HANDBOOK OF PSYCHIATRIC DRUGS

Lisa A. Burwell, MD

Current Clinical Strategies Psychiatry Associates

Publishing information for authors may be obtained by writing to:

Current Clinical Strategies Publishing
9550 Warner Ave, Suite 350
Fountain Valley, CA 92708-2822
Phone: 800-331-8227
Fax: 714-965-9401

Printed in USA ISBN 0-9626030-6-6

CONTENTS

Dedication

This book is dedicated to Ashley.
You bring us unending happiness and love.

ANTIPSYCHOTICS (NEUROLEPTICS)

Mechanism of Action: Dopamine postsynaptic receptor blockade; blockade and potentiation of norepinephrine.

Pharmacokinetics: After oral absorption, peak plasma levels usually occur within 2-4 hours. Undergoes extensive hepatic conjugation; 50% of neuroleptics are excreted via enterohepatic circulation; 50% of excretion is through the kidneys.

Pharmacology: Steady plasma levels may take up to 7 days.

Indications: Schizophrenia, schizophreniform disorder, schizo-affective disorder, mood disorders with psychotic features, drug induced psychoses, organic psychoses, acute mania; Tourette's syndrome.

Symptoms with good response to antipsychotics: Aggression, agitation, catatonic behavior, confusion, delusions, flight of ideas, grandiosity, hallucinations, hyperactivity, paranoid ideation.

SIDE EFFECTS:

Extrapyramidal Effects:

Akathisia: Most common in patients over 30 years of age. Restlessness, feeling a constant need to move about; agitation and anxiety, muscular tremor. Treat by administering an anti-Parkinsonism agent or reduce dose or switch to a low potency antipsychotic. If anticholinergics are not effective, benzodiazepines, clonidine, or propranolol (10 mg PO tid) may be effective.

Dystonia: Most likely to occur within the first week of treatment. Involuntary muscular contraction with sudden onset of rigidity and cramping; frequently involves the jaw muscles, as well as neck, tongue, face and back; hyperreflexia, oculogyric crises. More frequent with high potency antipsychotics. Treat with IV diphenhydramine (Benadryl); without treatment subsides in 24-48 hours after medication is discontinued.

Drug-Induced Parkinsonism: Usually occurs within first four weeks of treatment; more common in older patients. Rigidity begins in shoulders and then spreads to the rest of the body; stooped posture, drooling, shuffling gait, psychomotor retardation, masked face; tremor of the jaw, tongue and upper extremities and akinesia (inability to initiate movement); treat by switching to low potency antipsychotic and adding an anti-Parkinsonism agent.

Tardive Dyskinesia: Occurs after months to years of antipsychotic treatment, more frequent in older patients, in patients on long term antipsychotic treatment and in patients treated for affective disorders. Symptoms include tic-like movements of tongue, face and neck muscles, chewing movements; protrusion of tongue, excessive blinking and grimacing. Medication should be stopped if possible. No effective treatment exists. Use the lowest possible dose of antipsychotic medication. Irreversible in 25% of patients. The differential diagnosis of tardive dyskinesia includes Parkinson's disease, Huntington's disease, Sydenham's chorea; disorders are of movement commonly seen in schizophrenia.

Endocrinologic Effects: Reduction in testosterone levels, elevated serum prolactin levels, galactorrhea, amenorrhea, breast enlargement, reduced libido.

Antiadrenergic Effects: Lightheadedness, postural hypotension, tachycardia.

Anticholinergic effects: More common with more sedating antipsychotics; blurred vision, constipation, dry mouth; inhibition of ejaculation, urinary retention.

Antihistimatic effects: Sedation, weight gain, hypotension.

Neuroleptic Malignant Syndrome (NMS): Usually occurs during first week of treatment, but may occur after hours to months of treatment. More common in patients taking high potency antipsychotics (haloperidol, fluphenazine).

Risk factors: Dehydration, exposure to heat, exhaustion, organic mental disorder or poor nutrition.

Symptoms of Neuroleptic Malignant Syndrome: Catatonic like state of rigidity, delirium, fever, hyperthermia, diaphoresis, hypertension or hypotension, tachycardia and arrhythmias, elevated creatine phosphokinase; possible elevations in liver function and WBC; tremor, altered consciousness, myoglobinuria, renal failure, seizures and coma.

Treatment of Neuroleptic Malignant Syndrome: Medication should be discontinued immediately. Treat with cooling blankets, hydration, bromocriptine, dantrolene.

Other side effects: Fatigue, blurred vision, photosensitivity, sedation (use qhs schedule), lowered seizure threshold, skin rashes, EKG changes, reduced libido; delayed ejaculation, amenorrhea. Less commonly: Jaundice, agranulocytosis, eye or skin changes.

Contraindications: Narrow angle glaucoma, prostatic hypertrophy (urinary retention), liver disease.

Drug Interactions:

-CNS depression with all CNS depressants (including alcohol).

-Absorption of antipsychotics may be inhibited by antacids salts and anticholinergics.

-Anticonvulsant levels may be increased by antipsychotics.

-Anticholinergics decrease blood levels of antipsychotics and also increase sedative effects.

-Tricyclic antidepressants may reduce metabolism of antipsychotics; blood levels of tricyclics may be increased by antipsychotics.

-Digoxin absorption is increased.

-Barbiturates decrease blood levels of antipsychotics, may cause respiratory depression.

-ACE inhibitors may cause potentiate hypotension.

-Opiate narcotics cause potentiation of CNS sedation.

-Methyldopa can cause severe hypotension.

-Isoniazid can cause hepatic toxicity, encephalopathy.

Overdose: Death is rare from overdose of antipsychotics. Mesoridazine, pimozide and thioridazine are more dangerous and can cause heart block and ventricular tachycardia. CNS depression, hypotension, convulsions, fever, ECG changes, hypothermia or hyperthermia may occur.

Principles of Administration:

-Select an antipsychotic with a previous good response for the patient or family member.

-Adjust dose as patient improves.

-High potency antipsychotics tend to cause less anticholinergic symptoms

-Low potency antipsychotics (mesoridazine, thioridazine) slow cardiac conduction; patients with a history of cardiovascular disease should be treated with high potency antipsychotics.

-Antipsychotics are contraindicated in patients with hypotension, prostatic hypertrophy, narrow angle glaucoma.

-Postural hypotension is more common with low potency antipsychotics.

-When discontinuing antipsychotics the dosage should be slowly tapered.

-Aliphatic and lower potency antipsychotics reduce the seizure threshold significantly more than piperazines.

-Fluphenazine and molindone have been proven to cause less seizure activity than other antipsychotics.

-Elderly patients are more prone to CNS and cardiovascular side effects; use lower dose and monitor carefully.

-Use caution when administering to depressed patients; may worsen depression and increase suicide risk.

-Use caution in patients with impaired hepatic, respiratory or with cardiovascular disease.

-Use caution in patients with impaired renal function, and monitor renal function.

-Initially use divided dosages; administering before bedtime; may be used to reduce sedation and hypotension.

ANTIPSYCHOTIC AGENTS

BUTYROPHENONES

Haloperidol (Haldol)/ Haloperidol decanoate/Haloperidol lactate

Indications: Schizophrenia and other psychotic disorders, Tourette's syndrome.

Dosage Forms: 0.5, 1, 2, 5, 10, 20 mg tabs,
Haloperidol decanoate: 70.5/50 mg/ml, 141.0/100 mg/ml inj.
Haloperidol lactate: 5 mg/ml parenteral, 2 mg/ml conc.

Dosage: 2-5 mg IM q4-8h prn (haloperidol lactate) or 0.5-5 mg PO bid/tid, max 100 mg/day. Haloperidol decanoate IM: (switching from PO), 10 times previous dose once a month. PCP psychosis/acute psychiatric situations: haloperidol 2-5 mg IM every 30 minutes. Elderly: 0.5-2 mg PO bid/tid.

Therapeutic Blood Level: 5-20 ng/ml.

Advantages/Disadvantages: Lower incidence of sedation and hypotension than other antipsychotics; increased incidence of neuroleptic malignant syndrome; Haloperidol decanoate is a good choice for patients with a history of noncompliance.

Side Effects: Sedation, amenorrhea, weight gain, urinary retention, constipation, blurred vision, hypotension; dystonic reactions, akinesia, tardive dyskinesia, Parkinsonism, reduced libido, rashes, ECG changes, lowered seizure threshold, neuroleptic malignant syndrome.

Sedation: Moderate

Anticholinergic Effects: Less common

Hypotension: Less common

Extrapyramidal Effects: More common

Dosage equivalent to 100 mg Chlorpromazine (Thorazine): 1.6 mg

Potency: Low

Interactions:

-Fluoxetine may cause an increase in extrapyramidal reactions when it is taken in conjunction with haloperidol.

-Carbamazepine may decrease effect and level of haloperidol.

DIBENZODIAZEPINES

Clozapine (Clozaril)

Mechanism of Action: Blockade of dopamine at limbic receptors, adrenergic, cholinergic, histaminergic and serotonergic antagonist.

Indications: Refractory schizophrenia

Dosage Forms: 25,100 mg tabs.

Dosage: 25 mg qd/bid increase by 25-50 mg/day to 350-450 mg/day (in divided doses), then increase prn by up to 100 mg weekly (allow adequate time for dose to take effect and maintain at lowest possible dosage), max 900 mg/day. Usual dose: 300-600 mg daily. WBC with differential prior to beginning Clozapine and weekly during treatment, and for one month after Clozapine is discontinued. Patients should notify physician if weakness, fever, sore throat or flu symptoms develop. When discontinuing, taper over 2 weeks.

Advantages/Disadvantages: Risk of agranulocytosis; clozapine does not cause extrapyramidal side effects. Positive response in patients refractory to other neuroleptics.

Side Effects: Dizziness, seizures, orthostatic hypotension, sedation, gastrointestinal upset, fever, anticholinergic effects, cognitive impairment, hypersalivation, tachycardia; EEG and ECG changes; agranulocytosis, granulocytopenia, leukopenia. Increase in REM sleep, headache, tremor, restlessness, agitation.

Contraindications: Use with caution in patients with narrow angle glaucoma or prostatic enlargement and in patients with cardiac, hepatic or renal impairment.

Overdose: Drowsiness, delirium, coma, hypotension, excessive salivation, seizures, respiratory depression.

Sedation: More common

Anticholinergic effects: More common

Hypotension: More common

Extrapyramidal effects: Uncommon

Potency: **Low**

Dose Equivalent to 100 mg Chlorpromazine (Thorazine): 15 mg.

Interactions:

-Do not use in conjunction with any medication known to suppress bone marrow function.

-Potentiation of anticholinergic and antihypertensive medications.

DIBENZOXAPINES

Loxapine hydrochloride/Loxapine succinate (Loxitane, Daxolin)

Indications: Schizophrenia, other psychotic disorders.

Dosage Forms: Loxapine succinate: 5,10,25,50 mg tabs. Loxapine hydrochloride: 25 mg/ml concentrate, 1 ml/10 ml vial, 50 mg/ml parenteral.

Dosage: 10 mg PO tid, titrate to 60-100 mg day in divided doses; maintenance 20-60 mg PO qhs, max 250 mg/day or Loxapine HCL inj: 12.5-50 mg IM q4-6h or bid.

Advantages/Disadvantages: Drowsiness, seizures, increased incidence of AST/ALT liver function test abnormalities.

Side Effects: Sedation, constipation, dry mouth, blurred vision, hypotension. Reduced libido, weight gain, rash, photosensitivity, parkinsonism, dystonic reactions, akinesia, tardive dyskinesia, neuroleptic malignant syndrome, lowered seizure threshold.

Sedation: Less common

Anticholinergic Effects: Less common

Hypotension: Less common

Extrapyramidal Effects: More common

Potency: High

Dosage equivalent to 100 mg Chlorpromazine: 10 mg.

DIHYDROINDOLONES

Molindone (Moban)

Indications: Schizophrenia, other psychotic disorders

Dosage Forms: 5, 10, 25, 50, 100 mg tabs; 20 mg/ml concentrate.

Dosage: Adults: 5-25 mg PO tid-qid, increase as needed to a max of 225 mg/day (severe psychiatric conditions).

Advantages/Disadvantages: Molindone is less likely to precipitate weight gain; less likely to precipitate seizures. Less likely to cause amenorrhea and impotence.

Side Effects: Sedation, constipation, blurred vision, constipation, reduced libido, rashes, dry mouth; dystonic reactions, hyperactivity, photosensitivity, akinesia, parkinsonism, ECG changes; lowered seizure threshold, neuroleptic malignant syndrome, tardive dyskinesia.

Sedation: Less Common

Anticholinergic Effects: Common

Hypotension: Less common

Extrapyramidal Effects: Common

Potency: **Low**

Dosage equivalent to 100 mg Chlorpromazine (Thorazine): 10 mg

DIPHENYLBUTYLPIPERIDINES

Pimozide (Orap)

Indications: Tourette's syndrome

Dosage Forms: 2 mg tab.

Dosage: 0.5-1 mg PO bid, increase every other day as needed to a max of 0.2 mg/kg/day or 10 mg/day.

Advantages/Disadvantages: Increased incidence of cardiac effects, slowed cardiac conduction, high incidence of extrapyramidal effects.

Side Effects: Constipation, reduced libido, hypotension, sedation, weight gain, anticholinergic effects, rashes, galactorrhea, amenorrhea, dystonic reactions, akinesia, tremor, rigidity, ECG changes, tardive dyskinesia, parkinsonism.

Precautions: Use with caution in patient with a history of adverse reactions to anticholinergics, hypokalemia, hepatic or renal impairment.

Contraindications: Prolonged QT interval or in conjunction with medications that prolong the QT interval.

Sedation: Less common

Anticholinergic Effects: Less common

Hypotension: Less common

Extrapyramidal Effects: More common

Dose equivalent to 100 mg Chlorpromazine (Thorazine): 1-3 mg

PHENOTHIAZINES

ALIPHATICS

Chlorpromazine hydrochloride (Thorazine)

Indications: Schizophrenia and other psychotic disorders, mania, migraine headaches.

Dosage forms: 10, 25, 50, 100, 200 mg tabs; 30, 100 mg/ml concentrate; 10 mg/5 ml syrup; 25 mg/ml inj ; 30.75,150,200,300 mg sustained release caps.

Dosage: 10-50 mg PO bid/tid/qid increase prn (400 mg/day usually effective); Initial IM dose 25-50 mg, may be repeated q4-6h, may be increased slowly to a max of 800 mg IM/day. Switch to oral dosage as soon as possible.

Therapeutic Blood Level: 30-500 ng/ml

Advantages/Disadvantages: More likely to cause hypotension, anticholinergic side effects, agranulocytosis and allergic reactions.

Chronic use can cause bluish discoloration of skin; possibility of jaundice.

Side Effects: Hypotension, sedation, constipation, rashes, blurred vision, photosensitivity, weight gain, dystonic reactions, akinesia, lowered seizure threshold, tardive dyskinesia, Parkinsonism, agranulocytosis, neuroleptic malignant syndrome.

Contraindications: Blood dyscrasias, bone marrow depression. Use caution in patients with a history of cardiovascular, liver or renal disease.

Sedation: More common

Anticholinergic Effects: More common

Hypotension: More common

Extrapyramidal Effects: Less common

Potency: Low

Interactions:

- -Analgesics especially meperidine may increase hypotension and sedation.
- -Guanethidine effects may be decreased.
- -Valproic acid half life may be increased and its clearance decreased by chlorpromazine.

Triflupromazine (Vesprin)

Indications: Schizophrenia and other psychotic disorders (except depressive psychosis).

Dosage Forms: 10,20 mg/ml inj.

Dosage: Initially 60 mg IM, may be increased gradually to a max of 150 mg/day.

Sedation: More common

Anticholinergic Effects: More common

Hypotension: Common

Extrapyramidal Effects: Common

Dose equivalent to 100 mg Chlorpromazine (Thorazine): 25 mg

PIPERIDINES

Thioridazine hydrochloride (Mellaril)

Indications: Schizophrenia and other psychotic disorders.

Dosage Forms: Thioridazine HCl: 10, 15, 25, 50, 100, 150, 200 mg tabs, 30 mg/ml, 100 mg/ml concentrate. Thioridazine: 25,100 mg per 5 ml susp.

Dosage: Psychotic disorders: Initially: 25-100 mg PO tid increase prn to a maintenance of 100-400 mg PO bid, or 50-100 mg qid; max 800 mg/day.

Advantages/Disadvantages: More likely to cause sedation, seizures; high incidence of ventricular arrhythmias than other antipsychotics. Pigmentary retinopathy may occur rarely. Less risk of NMS and extrapyramidal effects than higher potency antipsychotics. Chronic use can cause bluish discoloration of skin.

Side Effects: Retrograde ejaculation; sedation, constipation, blurred vision, weight gain, reduced libido, rashes; seizures, dystonic reactions, akinesia, tardive dyskinesia, parkinsonism, neuroleptic malignant syndrome, retinopathy, gynecomastia, blood dyscrasias, jaundice.

Contraindications: Cardiovascular disease. Use caution in patients with seizure disorders.

Sedation: More common

Anticholinergic Effects: More common

Hypotension: More common

Extrapyramidal Effects: Less common

Dosage Equivalent to 100 mg Chlorpromazine (Thorazine): 100 mg

Potency: Low

Mesoridazine besylate (Serentil)

Indications: Schizophrenia and other psychosis, organic brain syndrome,

Dosage Forms: 10, 25, 50, 100 mg tabs; 25 mg/ml concentrate; 25 mg/ml inj.

Dosage: Psychosis: 25 mg IM (may repeat in one half hour) titrate as needed to a max of 200 mg/day, switch to oral dosage of 50 mg PO tid, max 400 mg/day.

Advantages/Disadvantages: Higher incidence of sedation and hypotension than other antipsychotics. Higher incidence of cardiac side effects than high potency antipsychotics.

Side Effects: Sedation, hypotension, dystonic reactions, akinesia, constipation, rashes, blurred vision, weight gain, reduced libido, ECG changes, tardive dyskinesia, neuroleptic malignant syndrome, Parkinsonism.

Sedation: More common

Anticholinergic Effects: More common

Hypotension: More common

Extrapyramidal Effects: Less Common

Dosage Equivalent to 100 mg Chlorpromazine (Thorazine): 50 mg.

Potency: Low

PIPERAZINES

Acetophenazine maleate (Tindal)

Indications: Schizophrenia and other psychotic disorders

Dosage Forms: 20 mg tabs

Dosage: Initially 20 mg PO tid, increase prn to 40-120 mg daily.

Side Effects: Sedation, dystonic reactions, akinesia, tardive dyskinesia, constipation, rashes, blurred vision, weight gain, reduced libido, Parkinsonism, ECG changes, tardive dyskinesia, neuroleptic malignant syndrome.

Sedation: Common

Anticholinergic Effects: Less common

Hypotension: Less common

Extrapyramidal Effects: More common

Fluphenazine hydrochloride (Prolixin)/ Fluphenazine decanoate (Prolixin Decanoate)/ Fluphenazine enanthate (Prolixin Enanthate)

Indications: Schizophrenia and other psychotic disorders.

Dosage Forms: Fluphenazine HCl: 1, 2.5, 5, 10 mg tabs, 5 mg/ml concentrate; 2.5 mg/5 ml elixir. 2.5 mg/ml inj. Fluphenazine decanoate/Fluphenazine HCl: 25 mg/ml inj.

Dosage: Fluphenazine HCl, 2.5-10 mg/day in divided doses, Maintenance: 1-5 mg PO qhs, max 20 mg/day **OR** 1.25 mg IM q6-8h, max 10 mg/day in divided doses. Elderly/adolescents -1-2.5 mg daily. Fluphenazine decanoate: 12.5-25 mg IM/SC q 4-6 weeks, max 100 mg. Fluphenazine enanthate: 25 mg IM/SC every other week.

Therapeutic Blood Level: 0.13-2.8 ng/ml

Advantages/Disadvantages: Less likely to cause seizures, long half life makes it difficult to titrate dose should side effects appear. Useful for noncompliant patients; lower incidence of ECG changes; Higher incidence of neuroleptic malignant syndrome with IM decanoate/enanthate.

Side Effects: Sedation, dystonic reactions, akinesia, constipation, rashes, blurred vision, weight gain, reduced libido, Parkinsonism, ECG changes, retinopathy, tardive dyskinesia, neuroleptic malignant syndrome; hypertension, insomnia, jaundice.

Contraindications: Subcortical brain damage. Use caution in renal, cardiovascular or hepatic dysfunction.

Sedation: Less common

Anticholinergic Effects: Less common

Hypotension: Less common

Extrapyramidal Effects: More common

Dosage equivalent to 100 mg Chlorpromazine (Thorazine): 1.2 mg

Potency: High

Perphenazine (Trilafon)

Indications: Schizophrenia and other psychotic disorders

Dosage Forms: 2,4,8,16 mg tabs; 16 mg/5 ml concentrate; 5 mg/ml inj.

Dosage: Initially: 8-16 mg PO bid/qid, max 64 mg/day; or 5-10 mg deep IM q6h, max 30 mg/day reduce slowly to maintenance of 4-8 mg PO tid/qid.

Therapeutic Blood level: 0.8-1.2 ng/ml

Advantages/Disadvantages: Less likely to cause seizures and ECG changes or hypotension. More likely to cause anticholinergic and extrapyramidal side effects.

Side Effects: Constipation, blurred vision, photosensitivity, hypotension, sedation; dystonic reactions, akinesia, Parkinsonism; rashes, weight gain, reduced libido, depression, ECG changes, lowered seizure threshold, jaundice, blood dyscrasias; retinopathy, tardive dyskinesia, neuroleptic malignant syndrome.

Contraindications: Hepatic and organic brain disease. Use caution in pulmonary, cardiac or renal impairment.

Sedation: Common

Anticholinergic Effects: Less common

Hypotension: Less common

Extrapyramidal Effects: More common

Dosage equivalent to 100 mg Chlorpromazine (Thorazine): 10 mg

Potency: Low

Trifluoperazine hydrochloride (Stelazine)

Indications: Schizophrenia and other psychotic disorders.

Dosage forms: 1, 2, 5, 10 mg tabs; 10 mg/ml concentrate; 10 ml vial; 2 mg/ml inj.

Dosage: Initially: 1-2 mg deep IM q4-6h (never less than 4 hours between doses), max 10 mg/day **OR** 2-10 mg PO bid/tid or 2-10 mg qhs. Maintenance: 15-20 mg daily.

Advantages/Disadvantages: Cardiac conduction changes are less likely with trifluoperazine than other antipsychotics.

Side Effects: Constipation, rashes, blurred vision, weight gain, photosensitivity, sedation, reduced libido, extrapyramidal effects, hypotension, seizures, neuroleptic malignant syndrome, tardive dyskinesia, jaundice, retinopathy.

Contraindications: Hepatic disease.

Sedation: Common

Anticholinergic Effects: Common

Hypotension: Less common

Extrapyramidal Effects: More common

Dosage Equivalent to 100 mg Chlorpromazine (Thorazine): 3 mg

Potency: High

Interactions:

-Methyldopa administered concurrently with chlorpromazine may cause marked elevations in blood pressure.

Prochlorperazine (Compazine)/ Prochlorperazine edisylate (Compazine)

Indications: Schizophrenia and other psychotic disorders.

Dosage Forms: Prochlorperazine: 5,10,25 mg tabs; 10,15,30 mg sustained release caps; 2.5,5, 25 mg supp. Prochlorperazine edisylate: 10 ml vial; 1,2 ml syringe; 2 ml amp; 5 mg/ml inj, 5 mg/ml syrup.

Dosage: Prochlorperazine: Initially: 5-10 mg PO tid/qid, titrate prn to a max of 100-150 mg/day **OR** prochlorperazine edisylate: 10-20 mg IM, repeated every 2 hours prn, max 4 doses (switch to oral dosage form as soon as possible) or 10-20 mg IM q4-6h.

Advantages/Disadvantages: Less likely to cause seizures, high incidence of extrapyramidal effects.

Side Effects: Sedation, constipation, rashes, blurred vision, dry mouth, constipation, salivation, diaphoresis, hypotension, weight gain, reduced libido, sedation, extrapyramidal effects, ECG changes, neuroleptic malignant syndrome.

Sedation: Common

Anticholinergic Effects: Less common

Extrapyramidal Effects: More common

Hypotension: Less common

Dosage Equivalent to 100 mg Chlorpromazine (Thorazine): 15 mg

Potency: High

THIOXANTHENES

Chlorprothixene hydrochloride (Taractan)

Indications: Schizophrenia and other psychotic disorders, behavioral disorders in mentally retarded.

Dosage Forms: 10, 25, 50, 100 mg tabs; 100 mg/5 mg concentrate; chlorprothixene HCl: 25 mg/2 ml inj.

Dosage: Initially: 25-50 mg PO/IM tid/qid, increase prn to a max of 600 mg/day.

Advantages/Disadvantages: Possibly, serious side effects are less frequent with chlorprothixene than other antipsychotics.

Side Effects: Neuroleptic malignant syndrome, constipation, rashes, blurred vision, hypotension, weight gain, extrapyramidal effects, ECG changes, altered thyroid function, retinopathy, hyperactivity.

Sedation: More common

Anticholinergic Effects: Common

Hypotension: Common

Extrapyramidal Effects: Common

Dosage Equivalent to 100 mg Chlorpromazine (Thorazine): 100 mg

Thiothixene/Thiothixene hydrochloride (Navane)

Indications: Schizophrenia and other psychotic disorders

Dosage Forms: Thiothixene: 1, 2, 5, 10, 20 mg caps. Thiothixene HCl: 5 mg/ml concentrate; 2 mg/ml solution for inj, 5 mg/ml inj.

Therapeutic Blood Level: 2-57 ng/ml.

Advantages/Disadvantages: Lower incidence of hypotension than other antipsychotics, NMS.

Dosage: Initially: 2-5 mg PO bid, max of 60 mg/day, maintenance of 10 mg PO bid/tid; thiothixene HCl inj: 4 mg IM tid/qid, max 30 mg/day. Switch to oral dosage a soon as possible.

Side Effects: Sedation, constipation, rashes, blurred vision, reduced libido, hypotension, lowered seizure threshold; Parkinsonism, dystonic reactions, akinesia, tardive dyskinesia, neuroleptic malignant syndrome, retinopathy.

Sedation: Less common

Anticholinergic Effects: Less common

Hypotension: Less common

Extrapyramidal Effects: More common

Dosage Equivalent to 100 mg Chlorpromazine (Thorazine): 5 mg

Treatment of Extrapyramidal Side Effects of Neuroleptics:

-Benztropine (Cogentin) 2 mg PO bid [0.5,1,2 mg].

-Lorazepam (Ativan) 1 mg PO tid [0.5,1,2 mg].

-Biperiden (Akineton) 2 mg PO qd/tid [2 mg].

-Clonazepam (Klonopin) 0.5 mg PO bid [0.5,1,2 mg].

-Trihexyphenidyl (Artane) 2-4 mg PO bid/tid [2,5 mg].

-Diphenhydramine hydrochloride (Benadryl) 25-50 mg PO bid/qid [25,50 mg].

-Amantadine hydrochloride (Symmetrel) 100 mg PO bid [100 mg].

ANTIDEPRESSANTS

TRICYCLIC ANTIDEPRESSANTS

Mechanism of Action: Blocks norepinephrine or serotonin reuptake.

Indications:

Clearly Indicated: Major depression; depression with anxiety and insomnia, bipolar disorder in conjunction with lithium; dysthymia, postpartum depression.

Sometimes indicated: Bulimia, anorexia, panic disorder, social phobia, somatoform pain disorder, generalized anxiety disorder; post traumatic stress disorder; premenstrual syndrome with depression (nortriptyline),

Symptoms most responsive to antidepressants: Fatigue, appetite disturbances, reduced libido, insomnia or hypersomnia, early morning wakening, frequent sleep disturbance.

Principles of Administration:

-Give anxious patients a sedating drug in the morning or before bedtime, give lethargic patients an activating drug in the morning.

-Evaluate past positive response of patient or family member to specific antidepressant medications. Consider side effects and choose a sedating or activating agent based on the patients type of depression.

-Limit quantities of medication available to depressed or suicidal patients.

-TCA's may precipitate manic episodes.

-Start with a low dose and increase until desired response is achieved or maximum dose is reached.

-Some TCA's contain sulfites or tartrazine (severe allergic reactions may occur), sensitivity is more common in asthmatics and in persons with aspirin allergies.

Benefits/Risks of Individual Agents

-Fluoxetine or trazodone are safer to prescribe to patients with suicide risk.

- -Desipramine is a good choice in patients complaining of sedation and anticholinergic effects.
- -Fluoxetine and imipramine are best for depression with panic attacks.
- -Sertraline, bupropion and fluoxetine are less likely to cause weight gain.
- -Sedation is common with doxepin and amitriptyline.
- -Nortriptyline, sertraline and bupropion are less likely to cause orthostatic hypotension.
- -Anxiety is common with desipramine, imipramine and nortriptyline.
- -Bupropion and fluoxetine may cause insomnia.
- -Amitriptyline, trimipramine and doxepin are often helpful in the depressed patient with insomnia.
- -Fluoxetine, trazodone, sertraline, and bupropion are best for patients with anticholinergic side effects.
- -Doxepin and amitriptyline are useful in patients with chronic pain.
- -Doxepin has antianxiety properties and should be considered in depression associated with anxiety disorders.

Anticholinergic Effects: Constipation, dry mouth, blurred vision, urinary hesitancy and retention; heat intolerance, increased intraocular pressure, prostatic hypertrophy. Signs of excess anticholinergic side effects include: agitation, confusion, restlessness, blurred vision, tachycardia, delirium, seizures, fever and dilated pupils.

Cardiac Effects: Postural hypotension, EKG changes, T-wave flattening, prolonged PR and QT interval, arrhythmias, palpitations, tachycardia, syncope. Contraindicated in patients with bifascicular block, prolonged QT interval and left bundle branch block.

CNS: Adverse CNS reactions include akathisia, ataxia, anxiety, agitation, difficulty with concentration and memory, coordination disturbances, headache, Fatigue, insomnia, nightmares, paresthesia, tremors.

Hematologic Effects: Agranulocytosis, anemia (clomipramine), eosinophilia, leukopenia, thrombocytopenia.

Autonomic Effects: Ejaculatory dysfunction, impotence (most common with clomipramine) and diaphoresis.

Drug Interactions:

-CNS depression with alcohol, anticonvulsants, sedatives, antihistamines or antipsychotics.

-Hypertensive crisis with MAO inhibitors.

-TCA plasma levels are increased by amphetamines, antipsychotics, estrogens, disulfiram, exogenous thyroid hormone, fluoxetine, glucocorticoids, oral contraceptives, salicylates or thiazides.

-TCA plasma levels are decreased by alcohol, barbiturates, carbamazepine, cigarette smoking, phenytoin, primidone, and rifampin.

-Hypotension is worsened by beta-blockers, clonidine, alpha-methyldopa, antipsychotics and diuretics.

-Clonidine effects are increased and hypertensive crisis has occurred when clonidine and TCA's were taken in conjunction with one another.

-Disulfiram can cause and increase in TCA levels and organic brain syndrome when it is coadministered with TCA's

-Antiparkinson agents, antihistamines and low potency antipsychotics increase anticholinergic effects.

-Phenytoin levels are increased

Signs/Symptoms of Overdose: Disorientation, delirium, agitation, hypertension, hyperpyrexia, hyperreflexia, myoclonus, nystagmus, pupil dilation, hallucinations, seizures (especially amoxapine and maprotiline), dry mouth, flushing, renal failure (amoxapine), urinary retention, CNS depression, coma, hypotension, intraventricular blocks, ventricular contractions, tachycardia, respiratory arrest.

TRICYCLIC COMPOUNDS

TERTIARY AMINES

Amitriptyline hydrochloride (Elavil/Endep)

Mechanism of Action: Blockade of serotonin (primarily) and norepinephrine reuptake.

Indications: Depression (especially endogenous).

Unlabeled uses: Bulimia nervosa, chronic pain.

Dosage Forms: 10, 25, 50, 75, 100, 150 mg tabs, 10 mg/ml inj.

Dosage: Depression: Initially: 50-100 mg PO qhs or 25 mg PO tid increase prn to 150 mg/day, max 200 mg/day; maintenance 50-100 mg PO qhs **OR** Initially: 20-30 mg IM tid/qid. Chronic pain: 25 mg PO qd/qid or 50-100 mg PO qhs.

Advantages/Disadvantages: Highly sedating (useful for insomnia), a first line- choice in patients with chronic pain, long half life; may be administered qd. High incidence of anticholinergic effects.

Side Effects: Sedation, constipation, dry mouth, blurred vision, weight gain; hypotension, GI upset (nausea), rash, headache.

Contraindications: Seizure disorder; within 14 days of a MAO inhibitor.

Time Delay for Therapeutic Effect: 3-4 weeks.

Therapeutic Level: 150-300 mg/ml

Anticholinergic Effects: Very common

Cardiac Effects: More common

Sedation: Very common

Hypotension: Common

Elimination Half Life: 10-50 hours.

Clomipramine hydrochloride (Anafranil)

Mechanism of Action: Blockade of serotonin (primarily) and norepinephrine uptake.

Indications: Obsessive compulsive disorder.

Unlabeled uses: Include treatment of panic disorder and chronic pain.

Dosage Forms: 25,50,75 mg caps.

Dosage: Initially: 25 mg PO qd (with food), increased over 2 weeks to 100 mg/day; then increased to max 250 mg/day, (maintenance doses may be given in a single dose qhs). Panic disorder 25 mg PO qd/tid or 25-75 mg PO qhs

Advantages/Disadvantages: High incidence of ECG changes; seizures, weight gain, and sexual disfunction. May precipitate manic episodes.

Side Effects: Constipation, dry mouth, blurred vision, urinary hesitancy, insomnia, GI upset, lowered seizure threshold, weight gain, esophagitis, sexual dysfunction (more common in males), dyspepsia.

Time Delay for Therapeutic Effect: 2-3 weeks.

Therapeutic Level: 80-100 ng/ml

Anticholinergic Effects: More common

Cardiac Effects: Common

Sedation: More common

Hypotension: Less common

Half Life: 19-37 hours.

Doxepin hydrochloride (Adapin, Sinequan)

Mechanism of Action: Blockade of serotonin (primarily) and norepinephrine reuptake.

Indications: Depression and anxiety associated with depression.

Unlabeled uses: Chronic pain, peptic ulcer, dermatologic uses.

Dosage Forms: 15, 25, 50, 75, 100, 150 mg caps, 10 mg ml Conc.

Dosage: Depression/Anxiety: 25-150 mg PO qhs or 25-50 mg PO bid/tid; maintenance: 25-50 mg PO tid or 75-150 mg PO qhs, max 300 mg/day.

Advantages/Disadvantages: Long half life; may use qd schedule; antianxiety properties, a first line treatment of chronic pain, frequent sedation (useful for insomnia).

Side Effects: Sedation or CNS stimulation, constipation, dry mouth, blurred vision, weight gain, urinary hesitancy, GI upset, hypotension, headache, rash. **Contraindications:** Glaucoma, history of urinary retention.

Time Delay for Therapeutic Effect: 3 weeks.

Therapeutic Level: 100-200 ng/ml

Anticholinergic Effects: Less common

Cardiac Effects: Common

Sedation: More common

Hypotension: Less common

Half Life: 8-24 hours.

Imipramine hydrochloride (Tofranil),Imipramine pamoate (Tofranil PM)

Mechanism of Action: Blockade of serotonin (primarily) and norepinephrine reuptake.

Indications: Depression (especially endogenous), enuresis.

Unlabeled uses: Panic disorder, bulimia nervosa, chronic pain.

Dosage Forms: 10, 25, 50 mg tabs, 25 mg/2 ml inj. Imipramine pamoate: 75, 100, 125, 150 mg caps.

Dosage: Imipramine hydrochloride: depression: 25-50 mg PO tid/qid, max 150 mg/day **OR** 25-100 mg IM/day (divided doses), switch to oral dosage as soon as possible. Imipramine pamoate: 75-150 mg PO qhs or 25-50 mg PO tid which may be increased to a max of 300 mg/day.

Elderly: 30-40 mg PO qhs, max 100 mg. Panic disorder: 25 mg PO qd/tid or 25-75 mg PO qhs. Chronic Pain: 25-50 mg PO tid or 75-150 mg PO qhs.

Advantages/Disadvantages: Long half life; may use qd schedule. Activating agent; anxiety may increase during first few weeks of treatment. Commonly used for depression in bulimic patients. Very effective in patients with depression and panic attacks.

Side Effects: Anxiety, CNS stimulation, constipation, dry mouth, blurred vision; insomnia, weight gain, GI upset (avoid taking on empty stomach), headache, rash, photosensitivity, urinary hesitancy.

Time Delay for Therapeutic Effect: 1-4 weeks.

Therapeutic Level: 150-350 mg/ml

Anticholinergic Effects: Common

Cardiac Effects: More common

Sedation: Common

Hypotension: More common

Half Life: 11-25 hours.

Trimipramine maleate (Surmontil)

Mechanism of Action: Blocking of serotonin (primarily) and norepinephrine reuptake.

Indications: Depression.

Dosage Forms: 5, 10 mg tabs; 25, 50, 100 mg caps.

Dosage: Initially: 25 mg PO tid/qid, increase prn to 50 mg PO tid or 75-150 mg PO qhs, 200 mg/day max. Maintenance: 50-100 mg/day PO qhs. Elderly: Initially 25 mg PO bid, increase prn to a max of 100 mg/day.

Advantages/Disadvantages: Sedating, long half life.

Side Effects: Heat or cold intolerance, sedation, constipation, dry mouth, blurred vision, urinary hesitancy; insomnia, GI upset (avoid taking on an empty stomach), tachycardia, weight gain, hyper or hypotension, rash.

Delay for therapeutic effect: One to four weeks

Therapeutic Level: 180 mg/ml

Anticholinergic Effects: Common

Cardiac Effects: Less common

Sedation: More common

Hypotension: Common

Half Life: 7-30 hours

SECONDARY AMINES

Amoxapine (Asendin)

Mechanism of Action: Blocking of norepinephrine (primarily) and serotonin (secondarily) reuptake.

Indications: Endogenous depressions, anxiety and agitation with accompanying depression.

Dosage Forms: 25, 50, 100, 150 mg tabs.

Dosage: Initially: 50 mg PO bid/tid, increase over one week to 100 mg PO bid/tid, max 400 mg/day in divided doses. Elderly: initially: 25 mg PO bid/tid, may increase to 50 mg PO bid/tid after 7 days, then prn up to 300 mg/day max.

Side Effects: Constipation, dry mouth, blurred vision, insomnia, sedation or CNS stimulation, seizures; dystonia, akinesia, parkinsonian reactions, urinary hesitancy, GI upset, weight gain, hypotension, rash.

Contraindications: Seizure disorder, myocardial infarction.

Advantages/Disadvantages: May take less time than other tricyclics for therapeutic effect. More likely to cause seizures.

Time delay for therapeutic Effect: 2-3 weeks.

Therapeutic Level: 200-500 ng/ml

Anticholinergic Effects: More common

Cardiac Effects: Less common

Sedation: Common

Hypotension: Less common

Half Life: 8 hours.

Desipramine hydrochloride (Norpramin)

Mechanism of Action: Blockade of norepinephrine (primarily) and serotonin reuptake.

Indications: Depression (especially endogenous).

Unlabeled uses: Bulimia nervosa.

Dosage Forms: 10, 25, 50, 75, 100, 150 mg tablets.

Dosage: 25-200 mg PO qhs or 25-50 mg PO bid/qid, max 300 mg/day; Elderly: 25-100 mg daily, max 150 mg.

Advantages/Disadvantages: Non-sedating, may worsen anxiety. Long half life; may use qd schedule. Lower incidence of anticholinergic effects than other tricyclics. Commonly used for depression in bulimic patients.

Side Effects: Anxiety, agitation, insomnia, CNS stimulation, weight gain, headache, rash; GI upset.

Time Delay for Therapeutic Effect: 3-5 weeks.

Therapeutic Level: 150-300 mg/ml

Anticholinergic Effects: Less common

Cardiac Effects: More common

Sedation: Less common

Hypotension: Less common

Half Life: 12-24 hours.

Nortriptyline hydrochloride (Pamelor)

Mechanism of Action: Blockade of norepinephrine (primarily) and serotonin reuptake.

Indications: Depression (especially endogenous).

Unlabeled uses: Panic Disorder.

Dosage Forms: 10, 25, 50, 75 mg caps, 10 mg/5 ml sol.

Dosage: 25 mg PO tid/qid, max 150 mg. Elderly: 10-15 mg PO bid/tid.

Panic Disorder: 25 mg PO qd/tid or 25-75 mg PO qhs.

Advantages/Disadvantages: Long half life, may use qd schedule. Activating agent; may worsen existing anxiety. Least likely to cause postural hypotension.

Side Effects: Anxiety, drowsiness, constipation, dry mouth, blurred vision, urinary hesitancy, CNS stimulation, headache, GI upset, rash.

Therapeutic Level : 50-160 ng/ml

Anticholinergic Effects: Common

Cardiac Effects: Common

Sedation: Common

Hypotension: Less common

Half Life: 18-44 hours

Protriptyline hydrochloride (Vivactil)

Mechanism of Action: Blockade of norepinephrine (primarily) and serotonin reuptake.

Indications: Depression.

Dosage Forms: 5, 10 mg tabs

Dosage: Initially 5-10 mg PO tid/qid may increase prn to a max of 60 mg/day. Elderly: 5 mg PO tid may increase prn.

Advantages/Disadvantages: Very low incidence of sedation. Long half life; may use qd schedule (qhs not recommended due to stimulant effects). Increased incidence of postural hypotension and tachycardia.

Side Effects: Constipation, dry mouth, blurred vision, insomnia, weight gain, CNS stimulation, hyper or hypotension, headache, rash, nausea, cardiovascular effects, urinary hesitancy.

Therapeutic Level: 100-200 ng/ml

Anticholinergic Effects: More common

Cardiac Effects: Common

Sedation: Less common

Hypotension: Less common

Half Life: 67-89 hours

TETRACYCLIC COMPOUNDS

Maprotiline hydrochloride (Ludiomil)

Mechanism of Action: Blocking of norepinephrine reuptake.

Indications: Depression, dysthymic disorder, bipolar disorder.

Dosage Forms: 25, 50, 75 mg tabs.

Dosage: Initially: 75-150 mg PO qhs increase gradually after 2 weeks by 25 mg prn; max of 225 mg/day, maintenance is 25-50 mg PO tid or 75-150 mg PO qhs. Elderly: 25 mg PO bid/tid or 50-75 mg PO qhs.

Advantages/Disadvantages: More likely to cause extrapyramidal effects and seizures.

Time Delay for Therapeutic Effect: 3-4 weeks.

Therapeutic Level: 200-300 ng/ml

Contraindications: Liver disease or seizure disorder.

Side Effects: Drowsiness, headache, CNS stimulation, anticholinergic effects, photosensitivity, edema, nausea, fatigue, rash.

Anticholinergic Effects: Common

Cardiac Effects: Less common

Sedation: Common

Hypotension: Less common

Half Life: 21-25 hours

Elimination Half Life: 26-60 hours.

ANTIDEPRESSANT/ANTIANXIETY/ANTIPSYCHOTIC COMBINATIONS

Chlordiazepoxide, Amitriptyline hydrochloride (Limbitrol)

Indications: Depression with anxiety

Dosage Forms: 5-12.5, 10-25 mg tabs

Dosage: Initially: one 10-25 mg tab PO tid max, may increase to a max of 6 tabs/day. Then reduce to lowest effective maintenance dose.

Advantages/Disadvantages: Useful in patients with chronic pain.

Contraindications: Recent myocardial infarction; within 14 days of a MAO inhibitor.

Interactions:

-Concurrent administration with a MAO inhibitor may result in hyperpyretic crises and death.

Perphenazine, Amitriptyline hydrochloride (Triavil, Etrafon)

Indications: Psychotic depression, anxiety, agitation.

Dosage Forms: Triavil: 2-10, 2-25, 4-10, 4-25, 4-50 mg tabs; Etrafon:
2-10, 2-25, Etrafon-A: 4-10, Etrafon-Forte 4-25 mg tabs.

Dosage: Etrafon: 1 tab PO tid/qid; max four 4-50 mg tabs/day. Triavil: 1 tab 2-25 or 4-25 tid/qid or 1 tab 4-50 PO bid.

Advantages/Disadvantages: Useful in patients with chronic pain.

Side Effects: Anticholinergic effects, extrapyramidal effects, drowsiness, dizziness.

SELECTIVE SEROTONIN REUPTAKE INHIBITORS AND OTHER ANTIDEPRESSANTS

Fluoxetine hydrochloride (Prozac) (Bicyclic)

Mechanism of Action: Inhibits serotonin reuptake.

Indications: Depression.

Unlabeled uses: Bulimia nervosa, obsessive compulsive disorder.

Dosage Forms: 20 mg tabs

Dosage: Depression: 20 mg PO qd increase as needed in divided doses up to 80 mg/day. Bulimia: 60-80 mg daily in divided doses.

Advantages/Disadvantages: No weight gain, insomnia, non-sedating, very few anticholinergic effects, long elimination half life; Best in patients with suicide risk, depression with panic attacks, or sensitivity to anticholinergic effects.

Side Effects: Restlessness, insomnia, rash, CNS stimulation, headache, anorexia and weight loss; impaired motor performance, anxiety, seizures, tremor, diaphoresis, nausea, vomiting, abdominal pain, diarrhea; precipitation of mania. If restlessness is a problem, combine with 0.25-0.5 mg clonazepam bid. Insomnia: reduce dose or treat with 25-50 mg trazodone at bedtime.

Contraindications: Discontinue if rash develops; pregnant or lactating women, use with caution in patients with impaired renal or hepatic function.

Overdosage: Symptoms include CNS stimulation, agitation, nausea and vomiting and seizures.

Interactions:

-Hypertensive crisis with MAO inhibitors.

Time delay for therapeutic effect: Two to five weeks.

Anticholinergic effects: Less common

Cardiac Effects: Less common

Sedation: Uncommon

Hypotension: Less common

Half Life: 7-9 days.

Elimination Half Life: 7-9 days.

Sertraline hydrochloride (Zoloft)

Mechanism of Action: Blocking of serotonin reuptake; blockade of dopamine and norepinephrine reuptake.

Indications: Depression.

Unlabeled uses: Obsessive/Compulsive disorder.

Dosage Forms: 50, 100 mg scored tabs.

Dosage: Depression/obsessive compulsive disorder: Initially 50 mg PO qd increase prn up to a max of 200 mg daily.

Advantages/Disadvantages: Less likely to precipitate weight gain, useful in patients with sensitivity to anticholinergic effects or orthostatic hypotension.

Side Effects: CNS stimulation, fever, back pain, hot flashes, thirst, decrease in serum uric acid, weight loss, diarrhea, nausea, abdominal pain, anxiety, insomnia, delayed ejaculation, dizziness, somnolence, tremor, dry mouth, agitation, rashes, syncope, chest pain, palpitations, headache, male sexual dysfunction.

Contraindications: Renal disfunction, severe hepatic disfunction, pregnancy and lactation; within 14 days of an MAO inhibitor.

Half Life: 24 Hours

Trazodone hydrochloride (Desyrel)

Mechanism of Action: Blocking of serotonin reuptake, potentiation of 5 - hydroxytryptophan

Indications: Major depression, particularly with anxiety or insomnia.

Unlabeled uses: Cocaine withdrawal, panic disorder, agoraphobia with panic attacks, aggressive behavior.

Dosage Forms: 50, 100, 150, 300 mg tabs.

Dosage: Depression: 50 mg PO tid, (should be taken with food) increase as needed by 50 mg every 3-4 days, max 400 mg/day in divided doses. Aggressive behavior: 50 mg PO bid (with tryptophan). May cause extreme sedation; qhs dosage may be necessary until patient adjusts to medication.

Advantages/Disadvantages: May produce sedation, minimal anticholinergic properties, relatively safe in overdose.

Therapeutic Level: 800-1600 ng/mcL

Time Delay for Therapeutic Effect: 2-4 Weeks

Side Effects: Drowsiness, dizziness, fainting (trazodone should not be taken on an empty stomach) fatigue, CNS stimulation, headache, nausea, vomiting, dry mouth, blurred vision, hypotension, syncope, priapism, impotence.

Contraindications: Trazodone hypersensitivity, recent myocardial infarction, pregnancy and lactation.

Anticholinergic Effects: Less common

Cardiac Effects: Common

Sedation: Common

Hypotension: Common

Half Life: 4-9 hours

Bupropion hydrochloride (Wellbutrin)

Mechanism of Action: Blockade of dopamine, norepinephrine and serotonin.

Indications for Use: Depression

Dosage Forms: 75, 100 mg tabs.

Dosage: Initially: 100 mg PO bid, maintenance: 100 mg PO tid, max 450 mg/day.

Advantages/Disadvantages: May be particularly useful in bipolar disorder, agitation, insomnia, weight loss, seizures. no anticholinergic effects, less cardiovascular toxicity and orthostatic hypotension than tricyclics, possibility for abuse due to stimulant properties.

Time Delay for Therapeutic Effect: 2-4 Weeks.

Side Effects: More common: CNS stimulation, dry mouth, constipation, agitation and insomnia , headache, nausea and vomiting, constipation, weight loss or gain, tremors, seizures (3-4 times more common than with other antidepressants), psychosis.

Contraindications: Seizure disorder, within 14 days of a MAO inhibitor.

Anticholinergic Effects: Common

Cardiac Effects: Less common

Sedation: Less common

Hypotension: Less common

Half Life: 8-24 hours

Paroxetine (Paxil)

Classification: Antidepressant

Mechanism of Action: Serotonin reuptake inhibitor

Indications: Depression, anxiety

Dosage Forms: 20,30 mg scored tabs.

Dosage: Initially: 20 mg PO/q am with food, then increased at 3 week intervals to a max of 50 mg daily. Elderly: Initially: 10 mg PO/q am with food, increase as indicated to 40 mg/day max.

Side Effects: Nausea, fatigue, somnolence, tremor, dry mouth, constipation, blurred vision, insomnia, decreased libido; dizziness, headache, weight loss or gain, sedation, anxiety, hypotension, rash, sexual disfunction, asthenia, manic episodes; palpitation, vasodilation, GI upset.

Advantages/Disadvantages: Less frequency of side effects than other antidepressants.

Contraindications: Within 14 days of a MAO inhibitor, use caution in suicidal and bipolar patients.

MONOAMINE OXIDASE INHIBITORS

Mechanisms of Action: Inhibition of monamine oxidase system (MAO), increase in epinephrine, norepinephrine, and serotonin.

Indications for Use: Atypical depression, major depression, dysthymic disorder, panic attacks, agoraphobia with panic attacks. Usually reserved for use in patients who have failed to respond to other antidepressants.

Principles of Administration:

-Use extreme caution when prescribing to suicidal patients.

-Patient should notify physician before taking any other medication (including nonprescription medications).

-Wait 7-14 days after discontinuation of MAO inhibitor before prescribing other medications.

-Teach patient to recognize signs of a hypertensive crises.

-Discontinue medication if headaches or palpitations occur.

-Tranylcypromine is a more rapidly acting agent with effects after 10 days.

-Manic episodes may occur in patients with bipolar disorder; psychosis may occur in patients with schizophrenia.

Side Effects: Orthostatic hypotension, hypomania, anxiety, headache, insomnia, impotence, dry mouth, agitation, dizziness, constipation, weight gain, seizures; GI upset (take medication with meals), muscle cramps (treat with pyridoxine 50-100 mg/day), urinary hesitancy, rash, liver damage (phenelzine, isocarboxazid).

Contraindications: Cardiovascular, renal or liver disease, severe hypertension, history of migraine headache; patients over 60 years of age.

Interactions with Foods:

Fruits: Canned figs, raisins, bananas, overripe fruit.

Vegetables: Fava beans (Italian green beans), sauerkraut, avocados, bean curd, soy sauce.

Dairy: Aged yogurt, strong cheeses, sour cream.

Meat Products: Liver, spoiled meat, fermented sausages (bologna, salami, pepperoni), meat tenderizer and extracts.

Fish: Dried, salted fish. Pickled or dried herring; caviar, shrimp paste.

Beverages: Beer, chianti/red wine, sherry any non-distilled alcohol.

Drug Interactions

- -Meperidine can cause hypotension and hypertension, fever, delirium, and death with MAOI's.
- -Tricyclic antidepressants can cause anxiety, disorientation, nausea, seizures, hypothermia, diaphoresis, tachycardia, coma and death.
- -Over-the-counter cold remedies and diet pills may precipitate hypertensive episodes, arrhythmias, headaches and convulsions.
- -Antipsychotics can cause extrapyramidal and hypotensive reactions.

Hypertensive Crisis: Occurs with tricyclic antidepressants, tyramine containing foods, adrenergic medications, amphetamines, cocaine, anorectics, dopamine, L-dopa, methyldopa, phenylephrine, pseudoephedrine, metaraminol, ephedrine, epinephrine, phenylpropanolamine, norepinephrine, meperidine (Demerol). Symptoms of hypertensive crisis: Headache, diaphoresis, mydriasis, hypertension, photophobia, tachycardia, bradycardia, angina, nausea, vomiting.

Treatment of Hypertensive Emergency

- -Phentolamine (Regitine) 5 mg IV then 0.25-0.50 mg IM q4-6h.
- -Nitroprusside sodium 0.25 -10 mcg/kg/min IV (50 mg in 250 ml of D5W), titrate to desired BP. Discontinue if acute fall in BP >30 systolic.

Overdose: CNS excitation, followed by CNS depression and cardiovascular collapse. Symptoms include anxiety, irritability, insomnia, restlessness, hypotension, weakness, sedation, dizziness, tachycardia, tachypnea, headache, coma, convulsions.

Isocarboxazid (Marplan)

Indications: Depressed patients who are refractory to tricyclic antidepressants or ECT, or when tricyclic antidepressants are contraindicated.

Dosage Forms: 10 mg tabs

Dosage: Initially: 30 mg PO qd then reduce to maintenance of 10-20 mg daily.

Advantages/Disadvantages: Hypertensive crises; use extreme caution in patients with impaired renal function.

Time Delay for Therapeutic Effect: 3-4 weeks.

Phenelzine sulfate (Nardil)

Indications: Atypical, nonendogenous or neurotic depression; depressions with phobic, hypochondriacal, anxiety features.

Dosage Forms: 15 mg tabs

Dosage: 15 mg PO bid, increase to 15 mg PO tid after three days; then by 15 mg weekly to 20 mg PO tid; max, 90 mg/day.

Advantages/Disadvantages: Hypertensive crises; possible pyridoxine deficiency; weight gain is common.

Time Delay for Therapeutic Effect: 3-4 Weeks.

Tranylcypromine sulfate (Parnate)

Indications: Major depression (reactive).

Dosage Forms: 10 mg tabs.

Dosage: 10 mg PO bid, increase to 15 mg PO bid after one week; then increase by 10 mg every 1-3 weeks to 50-60 mg/day; 60 mg/day max. When discontinuing medication should be tapered gradually.

Advantages/Disadvantages: Hypertensive crises; more stimulation than other MAO inhibitors, less likely to cause weight gain than other MAO inhibitors, Rapid onset (10 days).

Time Delay for Therapeutic Effect: 10 days

BENZODIAZEPINES

Mechanism of Action: Potentiation of gamma-aminobutyrate (GABA).

Indications: Insomnia, alcohol withdrawal, panic attacks, generalized anxiety disorders.

CNS/Psychiatric Side Effects: Sedation, impaired concentration, ataxia, drowsiness; paradoxical agitation, vertigo, depression, memory impairment, confusion.

GI Side Effects: Diarrhea, constipation, dry mouth, nausea, vomiting, anorexia.

Other Side Effects: Dependence and withdrawal, rash, allergic reactions

Symptoms of Withdrawal: Insomnia, irritability, tremor, agitation, abdominal discomfort, photosensitivity, seizures and psychosis.

Principles of Administration

- -Diazepam, prazepam, and chlordiazepoxide are long acting agents and may be given less frequently than short acting agents such as alprazolam, halazepam, oxazepam, and lorazepam.
- -Elderly patients and patients with medical conditions may require lower doses.
- -Diazepam is the best choice for rapid control of symptoms due to its rapid onset of action.
- -Lorazepam may be administered by intramuscular injection.
- -Short acting benzodiazepines have less potential for unwanted sedation.
- -Long acting benzodiazepines may have less withdrawal effects than short acting agents.
- -Periodically evaluate need for continuing treatment; not intended for long term administration.
- -Dose should be tapered when discontinuing medication.

Drug Interactions:

- -CNS depressants increase sedation.
- -Alcohol, disulfiram, valproic acid and isoniazid all reduce the metabolism of benzodiazepines.

-Estrogens and rifampin increase the metabolism of benzodiazepines.

-Antacids lower absorption, alcohol increases absorption.

-Cimetidine, disulfiram, estrogens, fluoxetine, isoniazid, ketoconazole, metoprolol, propranolol and valproic acid raise plasma levels of benzodiazepines.

-Levodopa's anti-Parkinson effect is reduced by benzodiazepines.

Overdose Symptoms: Ataxia, hypotonia, nystagmus, and coma.

Alprazolam (Xanax)

Indications: Anxiety disorders

Unlabeled uses: Depression, premenstrual syndrome.

Dosage Forms: 0.25, 0.5, 1, 2 mg tabs.

Dosage: Anxiety: 0.25-0.5 mg PO tid, max 4 mg/day; elderly 0.25 bid/tid. Panic disorder: 0.5-1 mg PO tid. Social phobia: 1-2 mg PO qid.

Advantages/Disadvantages: Dependence is common; abrupt discontinuation may result in withdrawal symptoms. Short acting (less potential for unwanted sedation).

Side Effects: Sedation, CNS depression, impaired concentration and memory, ataxia, drowsiness; hypotension, headache, paradoxical agitation, nausea, vertigo, seizures, tremors.

Interactions:

-Effects of digoxin may be potentiated when taken with alprazolam.

-Increase in levels of imipramine and desipramine.

-Potentiated by cimetidine and oral contraceptives.

Onset of Action: Moderate

Half Life: 12 hrs.

Duration of Action: Long

Chlordiazepoxide (Libritabs)/Chlordiazepoxide hydrochloride (Librium)

Indications: Anxiety disorders, alcohol withdrawal.

Dosage Forms: 5, 10, 25 mg caps and tabs; 100 mg powder for inj.

Dosage: Anxiety: 5-25 mg PO tid/qid; alcohol withdrawal/anxiety: 25-100 mg PO/IM q2-4h; elderly; 5 mg bid/tid/qid.

Advantages/Disadvantages: Dependence and withdrawal. Long acting agent; may be administered qd.

Side Effects: Sedation, impaired concentration, ataxia, paradoxical agitation, tolerance and dependence.

Interactions: Effects of levodopa are decreased. Serum levels of phenytoin are increased.

Onset of Action: Moderate

Half Life: 23-48 hrs.

Length of Action: Long

Clorazepate dipotassium (Tranxene)

Indications: Anxiety, alcohol withdrawal

Dosage Forms: 3.75 mg, 7.5 mg, 11.25, 22.5, 15 mg, scored tabs.

Dosage: 10 mg PO tid or 15 mg PO qhs, increase as needed to the usual effective dose of 15-60 mg/day; max 90 mg/day. Elderly: 7.5-15 mg daily in divided doses. Alcohol withdrawal, initially: 30-60 mg, increased by 30 mg on day 2, and reduced by 40 mg on day 3, then reduce by 10 mg daily.

Advantages/Disadvantages: Dependence and withdrawal.

Side Effects: Sedation, impaired concentration, ataxia, drowsiness; rash, headache, hypotension, tolerance and dependence, CNS depression; memory impairment; GI upset, blurred vision, dry mouth, tremor.

Onset of action: Moderate

Half Life: Approx 100 hrs.

Length of Action: Long

Diazepam (Valium)

Indications: Anxiety, acute alcohol withdrawal.

Unlabeled uses: Panic attacks.

Dosage Forms: 2.5, 10 mg, scored tabs, 5 mg/ml solution and inj.

Dosage: Anxiety: 2-10 mg PO bid/qid **OR** 2-20 mg IV (5 mg/min). Elderly 1-2.5 mg qd/bid. Alcohol withdrawal: 5-10 mg PO tid/qid first day, reduce to 5 mg tid prn and **OR** 5-10 mg IV/IM first dose, followed by 5 mg IV/IM q4h prn.

Advantages/Disadvantages: Long acting agent; may be administered qd; potential for unwanted sedation; dependence and withdrawal may occur.

Side Effects: Sedation, impaired concentration and memory, ataxia, drowsiness; hypotension, nausea.

Contraindications: Narrow angle glaucoma. Precautions: Liver or renal disease.

Onset of Action: Rapid

Half Life: 60 hours.

Duration of Action: Long

Interactions:

- -Theophyllines and rifampin may decrease effects of diazepam.
- -Valproate and fluoxetine (Prozac) may increase effects of diazepam.
- -TCA's may increase sedation.

Half Life: Long

Halazepam (Paxipam)

Indications: Anxiety disorders

Dosage Forms: 20, 40 mg tabs.

Dosage: 20-40 mg PO tid/qid, max 150 mg/day. Elderly: 10-20 mg PO qd/bid.

Advantages/Disadvantages: Long half life; less withdrawal effects, may be administered qd. Dependence and withdrawal.

Side Effects: Sedation, impaired concentration, ataxia, drowsiness; tolerance, rash, hypotension, paradoxical agitation, nausea, vertigo.

Onset of Action: Slow

Half Life: 48-50 hrs.

Duration of Action: Long

Flurazepam hydrochloride (Dalmane)

Indications: Insomnia

Dosage Forms: 15, 30 mg tabs

Dosage: 15-30 mg PO qhs.

Advantages/Disadvantages: May be administered qd; possible unwanted sedation. Dependence and withdrawal.

Side Effects: Elevations of liver function studies. Sedation, impaired concentration, blurred vision, ataxia, drowsiness; hypotension, paradoxical agitation.

Onset of Action: Fast

Half Life: approx 100 hrs.

Duration of Action: Long

Lorazepam (Ativan)

Indications: Anxiety

Dosage Forms: 0.5, 1, 2 mg tabs; 2,4 mg/ml inj.

Dosage: Anxiety: 0.5-3.0 mg PO bid/tid; Insomnia: 2-4 mg PO qhs. Elderly; 1-2 mg daily, divided doses.

Advantages/Disadvantages: Short acting, less potential for unwanted sedation. Dependence and withdrawal.

Side Effects: Impaired concentration and memory; ataxia, hypotension, paradoxical agitation, sedation, nausea, vertigo; tolerance and dependence.

Onset of Action: Moderate

Half Life: 12-15 hrs.

Duration of Action: Moderate

Oxazepam (Serax)

Indications: Anxiety disorders, anxiety in depressive disorders. Especially useful in older patients, and for alcohol withdrawal.

Dosage Forms: 10, 15, 30 mg caps; 15 mg tabs.

Dosage: Anxiety: 10-30 mg PO tid/qid; Elderly: 10 mg PO tid/qid. Alcohol withdrawal; 15-30 mg PO tid/qid.

Advantages/Disadvantages: Dependence and withdrawal.

Side Effects: Sedation, impaired concentration and memory; ataxia, hypotension, paradoxical agitation; nausea, vertigo; rash, tolerance and dependence.

Contraindications: Psychotic disorders.

Onset of Action: Slow

Half Life: 8 hrs

Duration of Action: Moderate

Prazepam (Centrax)

Indications: Anxiety disorders.

Dosage Forms: 5, 10, 20 mg cap, 10 mg tabs

Dosage: 10-20 mg PO tid **OR** 20-40 mg PO qhs; elderly: 10-15 mg daily in divided doses.

Advantages/Disadvantages: Dependence and withdrawal, potential for unwanted sedation.

Side Effects: Sedation, dry mouth, impaired concentration and memory, ataxia; hypotension, paradoxical agitation, tolerance and dependence.

Onset of Action: Slow

Half Life: Approx 100 hours

Duration of Action: Long

Estazolam (ProSom)

Indications: Insomnia

Dosage Forms: 1,2 mg tabs

Dosage: 1-2 mg PO qhs; elderly: 0.5-1 mg PO qhs.

Advantages/Disadvantages: Possible unwanted sedation.

Side Effects: Sedation, CNS depression, impaired concentration, ataxia, paradoxical agitation, tolerance and dependence.

Onset of Action: Moderate

Half Life: 10-24 hrs

Duration of Action: Moderate

Quazepam (Doral)

Indications: Insomnia

Dosage Forms: 7.5, 15 mg tabs.

Dosage: 7.5-15 mg PO qhs; elderly: 7.5 mg PO qhs.

Advantages/Disadvantages: Possible unwanted sedation. Dependence and withdrawal.

Contraindications: Sleep apnea.

Side Effects: Sedation, CNS depression, dry mouth, headache, impaired concentration, ataxia; hypotension, paradoxical agitation, tolerance and dependence.

Onset of Action: Moderate

Half Life: Moderate

Temazepam (Restoril)

Indications: Insomnia

Dosage Forms: 15, 30 mg caps

Dosage: 15-30 mg PO qhs; elderly: 15 mg PO qhs.

Side Effects: Sedation, CNS depression, ataxia, paradoxical agitation.

Advantages/Disadvantages: Less potential for unwanted sedation, early morning awakening may occur. Dependence and withdrawal.

Onset of Action: Moderate

Half Life: 10-12 hrs

Duration of Action: Short

Triazolam (Halcion)

Indications: Insomnia

Dosage Forms: 0.125, 0.25 mg tabs

Dosage: 0.125-0.25 PO qhs, 0.5 max; elderly or debilitated 0.125 mg PO qhs.

Advantages/Disadvantages: Short half life; good choice for patients with difficulty falling asleep; early morning waking may occur. Dependence and withdrawal. Possible rebound insomnia.

Side Effects: Sedation, CNS depression, ataxia, headache, paradoxical anxiety and agitation.

Precautions: Discontinue if agitation or excitement occurs.

Onset of Action: Fast to Moderate

Half Life: 2 hours

Duration of Action: Short

OTHER ANTIANXIETY AGENTS

Zolpidem tartrate (Ambien)

Mechanism of Action: Interacts with omega receptor of GABA

Indications: Insomnia

Dosage Forms: 5,10 mg tabs

Dosage: 10 mg PO qhs (7-10 days),

Advantages/Disadvantages: Less rebound and residual effects than other sedatives. Rapid onset of sedative effect.

Side Effects: Sedation, dizziness, amnesia, GI upset, nausea, vomiting.

Contraindications: Use with caution in patients with a history or drug abuse, depression; hepatic, respiratory or renal impairment.

Overdosage: CNS depression

Interactions: CNS depression with other CNS depressants (including alcohol).

Buspirone hydrochloride (Buspar)

Mechanism of Action: Blockade of serotonin, mild dopamine blockade, increases norepinephrine metabolism.

Indications: Anxiety.

Dosage Forms: 5, 10 mg tabs.

Usual daily dose: Adults 5-10 mg PO tid. Start with 5 mg PO bid and increase to 15-25 mg/day; 60 mg/day max.

Advantages/Disadvantages: Lack of sedation and dependence.

Side Effects: Headache, nervousness, fatigue.

Contraindications: Use with caution in renal or hepatic impairment.

Overdosage: Symptoms include: Drowsiness, dizziness, nausea and vomiting.

Interactions:

-Elevations in blood pressure with MAO inhibitors.

-Fluoxetine decreases effects of buspirone.

-Potentiation of haloperidol.

Half Life: 2-4 hrs.

BARBITURATES

Amobarbital (Amytal)

Mechanism of Action: Increases postsynaptic effects of gamma aminobutyric acid (GABA); decrease in postsynaptic release of neurotransmitters.

Indications: Hypnosis, insomnia, sedation

Dosage Forms: 15, 30, 50, 100 mg tabs; 65, 200 mg caps; 44 mg/5 ml conc; powder for inj.

Dosage: Sedation: 15-50 mg PO bid/tid. Insomnia: 50-200 mg PO qhs. Hypnosis: 100-200 mg PO qd.

Advantages/Disadvantages: Tolerance, dependance; extremely dangerous in overdose.

Side Effects: CNS depression, nausea, vomiting, diarrhea, dependence, withdrawal (taper gradually), nightmares. Impaired motor coordination.

Onset of Action: Moderate

Half Life: 8-42 hrs

Length of Action: Moderate

Butabarbital sodium (Butisol)

Mechanism of Action: Increases postsynaptic effects of gamma aminobutyric acid (GABA); decrease in postsynaptic release of neurotransmitters.

Indications: Sedation

Dosage Forms: 15, 30, 100, 150 mg tabs; 30 mg/5 ml conc.

Dosage: 15-30 mg PO tid/qid. Insomnia: 50-100 mg PO qhs.

Advantages/Disadvantages: Tolerance, dependance; extremely dangerous in overdose. Rarely used.

Side Effects: CNS depression, nausea, vomiting, diarrhea, dependence, withdrawal (titrate gradually), paradoxical agitation.

Onset of Action: Moderate

Half Life: 32-46 hrs

Length of Action: Moderate

Mephobarbital (Mebaral)

Mechanism of Action: Increases postsynaptic effects of gamma aminobutyric acid (GABA); decrease in postsynaptic release of neurotransmitters.

Indications: Sedation

Dosage Forms: 32, 50, 100, 200 mg tabs.

Dosage: 32 to 100 mg PO tid/qid.

Advantages/Disadvantages: Benzodiazepines are a safer choice. Tolerance, dependance; extremely dangerous in overdose.

Side Effects: CNS depression, drowsiness, nausea, vomiting, cramping, diarrhea; dependence, withdrawal (titrate gradually).

Onset of Action: Moderate

Half Life: 34 hrs

Duration of Action: Long

Pentobarbital (Nembutal)

Mechanism of Action: Increases postsynaptic effects of gamma aminobutyric acid (GABA); decrease in postsynaptic release of neurotransmitters.

Indications: Sedation.

Dosage Forms: 30, 50, 100 mg caps; 20 mg/ml conc; 2 ml amps; 20,50 ml vial; 50 mg/ml parenteral

Dosage: Sedation: 20 mg PO tid. Insomnia: 100 mg PO qhs.

Advantages/Disadvantages: Tolerance, dependance, extremely dangerous in overdose. Rarely used; other agents are a better choice.

Side Effects: CNS depression, drowsiness, nausea, vomiting, cramping, diarrhea; dependence, withdrawal (taper gradually).

Onset of Action: Short

Half Life: 15-48 hrs.

Duration of Action: Short

Phenobarbital

Mechanism of Action: Increases postsynaptic effects of gamma aminobutyric acid (GABA); decrease in postsynaptic release of neurotransmitters.

Indications: Sedation, insomnia

Dosage Forms: 8, 16, 32, 65, 100 mg tabs; 20 mg/5 ml elixir; 30, 60, 130 mg/ml inj.

Dosage: 20 mg PO tid/qid **OR** 100 mg PO qhs.

Advantages/Disadvantages: Tolerance, dependance, extremely dangerous in overdose.

Side Effects: Drowsiness, CNS depression; nausea, vomiting, cramping, diarrhea, dependence, withdrawal (taper gradually).

Onset of Action: Moderate

Half Life: 24-146 hours.

Duration of Action: Long

Secobarbital (Tuinal)

Mechanism of Action: Increases postsynaptic effects of gamma aminobutyric acid (GABA), decrease in postsynaptic release of neurotransmitters.

Indications: Insomnia

Dosage Forms: 100 mg tabs; 50, 100 mg caps; 50 mg/ml parenteral; 20 ml vials; 1, 2 ml syringe.

Dosage: 100 mg PO qhs.

Advantages/Disadvantages: Tolerance, dependance, extremely dangerous in overdose.

Side Effects: CNS depression, drowsiness, nausea, vomiting, cramping, diarrhea; dependence, withdrawal (taper gradually), nightmares.

Onset of Action: Short

Half Life: 20-35 hrs.

Duration of Action: Short

OTHER SEDATIVES

Chloral hydrate (Noctec)

Mechanism of Action: Cerebral depression

Indications: Insomnia

Dosage Forms: 250, 500 mg caps; 250 mg/5 ml, 500 mg/5 ml syrup, 325, 500 mg suppositories.

Dosage: 500 mg PO qhs. Not for long term use..

Advantages/Disadvantages: Tolerance and dependence.

Side Effects: GI upset, disorientation, headache, confusion, paranoia; ataxia.

Contraindications: Gastritis, duodenal or gastric ulcers; pregnancy and lactation, hepatic, cardiovascular or renal impairment.

Overdosage: CNS depression, hypotension, respiratory depression.

Meprobamate (Equanil, Miltown)

Mechanism of Action: CNS depressant, inhibits spinal reflexes.

Indications: Sedation, anxiety.

Dosage Forms: 200, 400, 600 mg tabs.

Dosage: 1.2 to 1.6 g/day in divided doses; max 2.4 g/day.

Advantages/Disadvantages: Tolerance, dependance, extremely dangerous in overdose.

Therapeutic Blood Level: 0.5 to 3 mg/dl.

Side Effects: Drowsiness, slurred speech, vertigo, CNS depression, weakness, paradoxical excitement, ataxia; dependence, withdrawal (taper gradually).

Overdosage: Sedation, CNS depression, arrhythmias, tachycardia or bradycardia, hypotension, respiratory depression.

Hydroxyzine hydrochloride (Atarax)/ Hydroxyzine pamoate (Vistaril)

Mechanism of Action: Analgesic, antihistaminic and muscular relaxant effects.

Indications: Anxiety

Dosage Forms: Hydroxyzine hydrochloride: 10, 25, 50, 100 mg tabs, 10 mg/5 ml syrup; 50 mg/ml inj. Hydroxyzine pamoate: 25,50,100 mg caps; 25 mg/5 ml susp.

Dosage: 50-100 mg PO/IM qid. Administer IM for acute states.

Side Effects: Dry mouth, drowsiness, tremor, convulsions, hypersensitivity reactions.

Overdosage: CNS depression, sedation.

Interactions: CNS depression with other CNS depressants.

PSYCHOSTIMULANTS

Indications: Attention deficit disorder, major depression.

Mechanism of Action: Stimulation of sympathetic nervous system by promotion of release of dopamine, norepinephrine and serotonin at presynaptic terminals, inhibition of dopamine, norepinephrine and monoamine oxidase.

Side effects: CNS stimulation, hypertension, dry mouth, anorexia, insomnia; palpitations, urticaria, psychosis, possible depression, GI upset.

Contraindications: Cardiovascular disease, hypertension, hyperthyroidism.

Interactions:

-Hypertensive crisis with MAO inhibitors.

-Increased effect with tricyclic antidepressants.

-Increased affect with other CNS stimulants.

Methylphenidate hydrochloride (Ritalin)

Mechanism of Action: Stimulation of sympathetic nervous system by promotion of release of dopamine, norepinephrine and serotonin at presynaptic terminals, inhibition of dopamine, norepinephrine and monoamine oxidase.

Indications: Narcolepsy, attention deficit disorder.

Dosage Forms: 5, 10, 20 mg tabs, 20 mg sust-release tabs, 5 mg/ml elixir.

Dosage: 10-60 mg per day in divided doses; Children over 6 years: 5 mg bid increase weekly, max 60 mg/day. Inform patient not to chew or crush sustained release preparations.

Advantages/Disadvantages: Dependance and tolerance.

Side Effects: Insomnia, CNS stimulation, anorexia, GI disturbances, hypertension, arrhythmias, tachycardia, psychosis, seizures.

Contraindications: Glaucoma, family history of Tourette's syndrome, severe anxiety.

Interactions:

-Guanethidine can be de-potentiated by stimulants.

-Increased affect with other CNS stimulants.

-Hypertensive crises with MAO inhibitors.

Pemoline (Cylert)

Mechanism of Action: Promotion of release of dopamine, norepinephrine and serotonin at presynaptic terminals.

Indications: Attention deficit disorder.

Dosage Forms: 18.75, 37.5, 75 mg tabs; 37.5 mg chewable tabs.

Dosage: Children over 6 years: 37.5 mg increased weekly by 18.75 mg; max 112.5 mg daily.

Advantages/Disadvantages: Dependance and tolerance, long half life; may use qd schedule.

Side effects: CNS stimulation, anorexia, insomnia, headache, rash. GI upset.

Interactions:

-Increased affect with other CNS stimulants.

-Hypertensive crises with MAO inhibitors.

LITHIUM CARBONATE

Mechanism of Action: Alteration of sodium levels and transport; increase in norepinephrine reuptake.

Indications: Bipolar disorder, cyclothymia; possibly schizophreniform and schizoaffective disorder.

Principles of Administration:

Labs Before Administering Lithium:

-CBC, BUN, serum creatinine, thyroid function tests, urinalysis, electrolytes; potassium, sodium, fasting glucose. ECG for patients over 40 years old.

-Start lithium at 300 mg PO bid/tid increase by 300 mg daily to therapeutic blood level of 1.2-1.4 mEq/L.

-After initiating therapy monitor lithium level weekly; after steady state is reached, monitor every 2 months.

-Maintenance blood level is 0.5-1.0 mEq/L.

-Monitor renal and thyroid function.

-Antipsychotics may be used in conjunction with lithium until therapeutic levels are reached.

-Advise patient to maintain adequate fluid intake.

Dosage: Starting dose 300 mg tid; increase dose based on blood level. An ideal blood level is 1.0-1.2 mMol/L.

Side Effects:

Central Nervous System: Headache, transient muscle weakness, lethargy, slurred speech, tremor.

Tremor: Treat by decreasing dose, and if necessary add propranolol 20-60 mg per day; start at 10-20 mg bid and increasing prn; or atenolol 50 mg per day.

Gastrointestinal Side Effects: Diarrhea, nausea, vomiting, anorexia, bloating, cramps, abdominal pain. Treat by giving smaller doses more often.

Endocrinologic Side Effects: Hypothyroidism, hyperthyroidism, goiter; hyperglycemia. Check thyroid function tests at least once every six months. Hypothyroidism can be treated with levothyroxine.

Renal: Thirst, polyuria, polydipsia; diabetes insipidus which can be treated with hydrochlorothiazide 50 mg daily or amiloride 5-10 mg/day.
Cardiac: Myocarditis, sinoatrial or atrioventricular block, T wave flattening or inversion; arrhythmias, bradycardia, sinus node dysfunction, syncope, QRS widening, hypotension.
Dermatologic: Folliculitis, acne, psoriasis; rarely alopecia and exfoliative dermatitis.
Contraindications: Pregnancy and lactation; patients with a history of myocardial infarction. Use extreme caution in patients with hypothyroidism, cardiovascular or renal impairment.
Drug Interactions:

-Lithium levels may be increased by thiazides, amiloride, ethacrynic acid, furosemide, ibuprofen, tetracyclines, piroxicam, mefenamic acid, indomethacin, sulindac, tetracycline, triamterene, spironolactone, methyldopa, metronidazole.

-Lithium levels may be lowered by calcium channel blockers, valproate, theophylline, diuretics.

-Renal toxicity has been reported with the combination of metronidazole and lithium.

-Potassium iodine increases incidence of goiter and hypothyroidism.

-Lithium excretion is increased by aminophylline.

Lithium Levels:

Therapeutic Lithium Levels	Mild to Moderate Toxicity	Moderate to Severe Toxicity	Severe Toxicity Over 2.5 mEq./L
0.6-1.5 mEq./L	1.5-2.0 mEq./L	2.0-2.5 mEq./L	

-Antipsychotics increase neurotoxic effects of lithium.

-Effects of tricyclic antidepressants may be increased by lithium.

Overdose/Intoxication: Precipitated by sodium depletion, dehydration and renal disfunction. Signs/symptoms of overdose: nausea, vomiting, renal failure, confusion, incoordination, difficulty concentrating, dysarthria, tremor, ataxia, delirium, seizures, coma.

ANTICONVULSANTS

Carbamazepine (Tegretol)

Mechanism of Action: Reduction of synaptic responses.

Indications: Acute mania, bipolar disorder, cyclothymia, schizoaffective disorder.

Dosage Forms: 100, 200 mg tabs.

Dosage: 800-1200 mg/day. Start at 200 mg per day and increase by 200 mg every 3-4 days until blood level of 4-12 mg/ml. Administer bid with meals.

Labs: Before starting carbamazepine: Obtain complete history and physical, CBC, liver and renal function tests. Continue to monitor CBC and liver function.

Side Effects: Sedation, blurred vision, nausea, GI upset; ataxia, vertigo, dysarthria; rash, tremor, delayed cardiac conduction, arrhythmias, hepatitis, aplastic anemia.

Contraindications: Pregnancy and lactation, within 14 days of a MAO inhibitor. Use with caution in patients with glaucoma; patients with cardiac, hepatic, or renal impairment.

Principles of Administration:

- -Monitor blood levels, liver function, urinalysis, and BUN. Less frequently monitor CBC, WBC with differential and platelet count.
- -Thyroid function tests may be altered.

Overdosage: Restlessness, seizures, CNS depression, ataxia, sedation, mydriasis, nystagmus. respiratory depression, hypotension or hypertension, tachycardia, nausea, vomiting.

Interactions:

- -Carbamazepine levels are increased by cimetidine, diltiazem, erythromycin, isoniazid, nicotinamide, valproic acid, propoxyphene and verapamil.
- -Carbamazepine levels are decreased by phenytoin, primidone and phenobarbital.

-Carbamazepine decreases effects of phenytoin, warfarin, ethosuximide; clonazepam, valproic acid, haloperidol and cyclic antidepressants.

-Effects of clonazepam are reduced by carbamazepine.

-Digitalis may produce bradycardia when administered in conjunction with carbamazepine.

-MAO inhibitors should not be administered within 14 days of carbamazepine.

-Theophylline is potentiated and potentiates effects of carbamazepine.

Half Life: 25-65 hours

Clonazepam (Klonopin)

Indications: Bipolar disorder, panic disorder, anxiety

Dosage Forms: 0.5, 1, 2 mg tabs.

Dosage: 2 mg qd/tid. When discontinuing, taper dosage to avoid withdrawal.

Therapeutic Blood Level: 20-80 ng/ml.

Advantages/Disadvantages: Addictive, withdrawal (status epilepticus, diarrhea and vomiting).

Side Effects: Sedation, ataxia, GI upset, hypersalivation.

Contraindications: Liver damage.

Onset of Action: Moderate

Half Life: 18-50 hours

Duration of Action: Moderate

Valproic acid (Depakene) and Divalproex (Depakote)

Mechanism of Action: Potentiation of postsynaptic gamma aminobutyric acid.

Indications: Acute mania, bipolar disorder

Dosage Forms: Depakene: 250 mg caps; 250 mg/5 ml syrup. Depakote: 125,250,500 mg tabs, 125 mg caps.

Dosage: 250 mg PO bid/tid, increase as tolerated to blood level of 46-102 mcg/ml; administration with food will decrease GI upset; qhs dosing will reduce sedation; should not be crushed or chewed.

Therapeutic Blood Level: 50-100 mcg/ml.

Side Effects: CNS depression, elevations of aminotransferase, hepatitis, hyperammonemia; GI upset, weight gain, drowsiness; ataxia, headache, rash.

Contraindications: Liver disease

Overdosage: Restlessness, hallucinations, coma.

Interactions:

-Increase in effect of MAOI's, phenobarbital and primidone; decrease in effects of carbamazepine.

-Toxicity of clonazepam is increased.

-Ethosuximide levels may be decreased.

-Potentiation of phenytoin and valproic acid.

-Chlorpromazine and cimetidine decrease clearance and increase life of valproic acid.

Half Life: 10 hours

ANTIPARKINSONIAN AND OTHER AGENTS

Amantadine hydrochloride (Symmetrel)

Mechanism of Action: Increases dopamine release.

Indications: Neuroleptic induced parkinsonism and dystonic reactions.

Dosage Forms: 100 mg caps; 50/5 ml syrup.

Dosage: 100 mg PO tid.

Advantages/Disadvantages: May cause insomnia.

Side effects: Nausea, dry mouth, blurred vision, constipation, anorexia, hypotension; dizziness, anxiety, insomnia, irritability, impaired concentration.

Contraindications: Seizure disorder, liver disease.

Interactions:

-Increased potency of CNS stimulants.

-Potentiation of anticholinergic effects of other anticholinergic medications.

Benztropine mesylate (Cogentin)

Mechanism of Action: Reduction of central cholinergic activity; increase in length of dopamine action.

Indications: Neuroleptic induced Parkinsonism, dystonic reactions.

Dosage Forms: 1, 2 mg tabs; 1 mg/ml ampules.

Dosage: 1-2 mg PO bid/tid **OR** 1-2 mg IM; max 6 mg/day.

Advantages/Disadvantages: Low incidence of adverse effects.

Side effects: Drowsiness, dry mouth, blurred vision, nausea, weakness, confusion; constipation, sedation, drowsiness, depression, psychosis.

Contraindications: Glaucoma, prostatic hypertrophy, myasthenia gravis, duodenal or pyloric obstruction.

Interactions:

-Increase anticholinergic effects with other anticholinergic medications.

Biperiden (Akineton)

Mechanism of Action: Reduction of central cholinergic activity; increase in length of dopamine action.

Indications: Neuroleptic induced Parkinsonism, dystonic reaction to neuroleptics.

Dosage Forms: 2 mg tabs, 1 mg/ml parenteral.

Dosage: 2 mg PO qd/tid.

Advantages/Disadvantages: Tolerance

Side Effects: Anticholinergic and antihistaminic effects; GI upset, depression, hypotension.

Contraindications: Glaucoma, prostatic hypertrophy, myasthenia gravis, duodenal or pyloric obstruction.

Interactions:

-Increased anticholinergic effects of with other anticholinergic medications.

Bromocriptine (Parlodel)

Mechanism of Action: Dopamine stimulation.

Indications: Parkinsonian syndrome, tardive dyskinesia.

Dosage Forms: 2.5 mg tabs; 5 mg tabs.

Dosage: Neuroleptic malignant syndrome: 2.5 mg PO bid/qid; Parkinsonian: 1.25 mg bid.

Side Effects: Fatigue, headaches, dry mouth, GI upset, hypotension, rash, drowsiness; elevated SGOT, SGPT, GGT, BUN, livedo reticularis, arrhythmias, hallucinations, confusion.

Contraindications: Impaired liver or renal function.

Interactions:

-Effects of bromocriptine may be reduced with phenothiazines or griseofulvin.

Diphenhydramine (Benadryl)

Mechanism of Action: Central anticholinergic activity, increase in dopamine action.

Indications: Neuroleptic induced Parkinsonism, dystonic reactions.

Dosage Forms: 25, 50 mg caps; 12.5/5 ml elixir; 10 mg/ml parenteral; 1 ml amp.

Dosage: 25-50 mg PO tid/qid or 10-100 mg Deep IM/IV max 400 mg/day.

Advantages/Disadvantages: Sedation

Side Effects: Blurred vision, dry mouth, irritability, insomnia, CNS depression; nausea, vomiting, constipation, sedation, gastritis, hypotension.

Contraindications: Narrow angle glaucoma, prostatic hypertrophy, pregnancy and lactation.

Interactions:

-CNS depression with CNS depressants.

-Increase in blood levels of phenytoin.

Procyclidine (Kemadrin)

Mechanism of Action: Central anticholinergic activity, increase in dopamine action.

Indications: Neuroleptic induced Parkinsonism, dystonic reactions.

Dosage Forms: 5 mg tabs.

Dosage: Initially: 2.5 mg PO tid, increase prn up to 5 mg tid/qid; 20 mg/day max.

Side Effects: Weakness, nausea, vomiting, anticholinergic effects, rash, tachycardia, urinary retention, delirium, heat stroke.

Contraindications: Glaucoma, prostatic hypertrophy, myasthenia gravis, duodenal or pyloric obstruction.

Trihexyphenidyl hydrochloride (Artane)

Mechanism of Action: Central anticholinergic activity, increase in length of dopamine action.

Indications: Neuroleptic induced Parkinsonism, dystonic reactions.

Dosage Forms: 2, 5 mg tabs; 5 mg caps.

Dosage: Initially 1 mg PO qd, increase prn up to 5 mg qd-tid; max 15 mg/day.

Advantages/Disadvantages: High incidence of anticholinergic and antihistaminic side effects.

Side Effects: Blurred vision, dry mouth, constipation, nausea, vomiting; weakness, tachycardia, weakness, restlessness, agitation, insomnia, tachycardia, urinary retention, delirium, hallucinations, heat stroke.

Contraindications: Glaucoma, myasthenia gravis, duodenal or pyloric obstruction.

Interactions: Increased anticholinergic effects with other anticholinergics.

Dantrolene (Dantrium)

Indications: Neuroleptic malignancy syndrome.

Dosage Forms: 25, 50, 100 mg caps; 20 mg parenteral.

Dosage: 50-200 mg PO daily.

Side Effects: Depression, weakness, drowsiness, slurred speech, dizziness, confusion, nausea, GI upset.

Contraindications: Liver disease, elevation of liver enzymes.

Disulfiram (Antabuse)

Indications: Alcoholism

Dosage Forms: 250, 500 mg tabs.

Dosage: 250-500 mg PO qd.

Side Effects: Fatigue, headache, impotence, acne, rash, irritability, insomnia, confusion, hepatitis. Less commonly: peripheral neuropathy, delirium and psychosis. If alcohol is consumed, headache, nausea, vomiting, pallor, thirst, diaphoresis, chest pain, anxiety, blurred vision; respiratory depression, arrhythmias, heart failure, seizures and death may occur.

Contraindication: Cardiovascular disease, psychosis, recent use of alcohol.

Interactions:

-Severe adverse reaction with alcohol consumption.

-Anticoagulant effects are increased with disulfiram.

-Theophyllines are potentiated.

-Metronidazole may precipitate a psychosis when administered in conjunction with disulfiram.

-Phenytoin levels are increased significantly.

-CNS depression with benzodiazepines.

-Isoniazid may cause behavioral changes.

-Tricyclics may cause organic brain syndrome when they are taken in conjunction with disulfiram.

INVESTIGATIONAL AGENTS

Dothiepin hydrochloride (Prothiaden)

Classification: Cyclic antidepressant

Mechanism of Action: Increased noradrenergic transmission, inhibition of serotonin uptake.

Indications: Depression

Efficiency in Clinical Trials: Dothiepin appears to be comparable to other tricyclic antidepressants in the treatment of depression and comparable to benzodiazepines in the treatment of associated anxiety.

Advantages/Disadvantages: Low incidence of anticholinergic effects.

Side Effects: Drowsiness, dry mouth, GI disturbances, tremor, dizziness, sweating; tremor, insomnia, weight gain, blurred vision, palpitations, headache.

Fluvoxamine (Floxyfral)

Classification: Cyclic antidepressant

Mechanism of Action: Inhibits reuptake of serotonin.

Indications: Major depression, obsessive-compulsive disorder, panic attacks.

Efficiency in Clinical Trials: Fluvoxamine appears to be comparable to imipramine, desipramine, imipramine in the treatment of depression.

Dosage: 50-300 mg daily

Advantages/Disadvantages: Useful in patients unable to tolerate tricyclics.

Side Effects: Nausea and vomiting, constipation, headache, dry mouth; agitation, somnolence, tremor, agitation, dizziness, syncope, manic episodes, insomnia, anorexia.

Interactions

-Propranolol and warfarin are potentiated by fluvoxamine

-Hypotensive and bradycardic effects are increased.

Gepirone hydrochloride

Classification: Antidepressant, anxiolytic; similar to buspirone.

Mechanism of Action: Serotonin antagonist

Indications: Depression, anxiety

Efficiency in Clinical Trials: Effective for anxiety and depression

Dosage: 25-75 mg daily

Advantages/Disadvantages: Delay for effect (2-3 weeks); non addictive.

Side Effects: Nausea, headache, dizziness, weakness and sedation.

Nitrazepam (Mogadon)

Classification: Benzodiazepine

Indications: Anxiety

Efficiency in Clinical Trials: Similar to other benzodiazepines.

Advantages/Disadvantages: Long elimination half life (30 hours).

Side Effects: Drowsiness, dizziness, fatigue, lethargy, nightmares, agitation, insomnia, rash, GI disturbances, headache.

Clobazam (Frisium)

Classification: Benzodiazepine.

Indications: Anxiety

Efficiency in Clinical Trials: Similar to other benzodiazepines.

Advantages/Disadvantages: Long elimination half life (18 hours).

Side Effects: Dizziness, drowsiness, weakness, weight gain, syncope, hypotension, dry mouth, headache, and GI disturbances.

Remoxipride (Roxiam)

Classification: Antipsychotic

Mechanism of Action: Dopamine antagonist, dopamine receptor blockade.

Indications: Psychosis, schizophrenia, acute mania

Efficiency in Clinical Trials: Appears to be as effective as other antipsychotics in treating schizophrenia.

Dosage: 150-600 mg daily

Advantages/Disadvantages: Possibly lower incidence of side effects (dry mouth, insomnia, sedation).

Side Effects: Same as other antipsychotics but less frequent.

TREATMENT OF AFFECTIVE DISORDERS

MAJOR DEPRESSION

Tricyclics

-Imipramine (Tofranil) 50-150 mg PO qhs or 25-100 mg PO qd/tid, max 300 mg/day or up to 100 mg/day IM (divided doses) [10,25,50 mg].OR

-Trimipramine (Surmontil) Initially: 25 mg PO tid, increase prn to a max of 200 mg/day [25,50,100 mg].

-Desipramine (Norpramin) 25-200 mg PO qhs or 25-100 mg PO qd/tid; max 300 mg/day [10,25,50,75,100 mg].**OR**

Other Antidepressants

-Bupropion (Wellbutrin) Initially 100 mg PO bid, increase to 100 mg PO tid after 4 days; max 450 mg/day; 150 mg/single dose [75,100 mg].OR

-Fluoxetine (Prozac) 20 mg PO qd up to 80 mg day (divided doses) [20 mg].**OR**

-Trazodone (Desyrel) Initially: 50 mg PO tid, increase by 50 mg every four days as needed; max 400 mg/day [50,100,150,300 mg].

MAO Inhibitors

-Phenelzine (Nardil) Initially: 15 mg PO tid, increase as tolerated to 60 mg daily. Then after a month to maintenance of 15-30 mg daily, max 90 mg/day [15 mg]. **OR**

-Isocarboxazid (Marplan) 10-30 mg PO qd or 10 mg PO qd/tid, max 3 mg/day [10 mg] **OR** Maintenance 10-20 mg daily.

-Tranylcypromine (Parnate) 10 mg PO tid, max 60 mg/day [10 mg].**OR**

DEPRESSION WITH INSOMNIA

-Doxepin (Sinequan) 25-50 mg qd increase to 75-150 mg qd as needed, max 300 mg/day [10,25,50,75,100,150 mg].**OR**

-Amitriptyline (Elavil) 75 mg qd increase as needed, max 150 mg/day or Initially: 10-30 mg IM tid/qid, switch to oral dosage [10,25,50,75,100,150 mg].

DEPRESSION WITH ANXIETY

Tricyclics

-Doxepin (Sinequan) 25-50 mg qd increase to 75-150 mg qd as needed, max 300 mg/day, [10,25,50,75,100,150 mg].

-Imipramine (Tofranil) 75 mg qd increase as needed to a maximum of 200 mg/day or up to 100 mg/day IM (divided doses) [10,25,50 mg].OR

MAO inhibitors (Especially useful in depression with anxiety and panic).

-Tranylcypromine (Parnate) 10 mg PO tid, max 60 mg/day [10 mg].

-Isocarboxazid (Marplan) 10-30 mg PO qd or 10 mg PO tid, max 30 mg/day [10 mg].

Other

-Alprazolam (Xanax) 0.25-2 mg PO tid/qid, max 8 mg/day [0.25,0.5,1,2 mg tabs].

-Oxazepam (Serax) 15-30 mg PO tid, [10,15,30 mg]

ATYPICAL DEPRESSION

MAO INHIBITORS

-Isocarboxazid (Marplan) 10-30 mg PO qd or 10 mg PO qd/tid, max 30 mg/day [10 mg].

-Tranylcypromine (Parnate) 10 mg PO tid, max 60 mg/day [10 mg].

Tricyclics

-Trimipramine (Surmontil) 25 mg PO tid max, 200 mg/day [25,50,100 mg].

-Imipramine (Tofranil) 50-150 mg PO qhs, max 200 mg/day or up to 100 mg IM/day (divided doses) [10,25,50 mg].

DYSTHYMIA

Tricyclics:

-Trazodone (Desyrel) 50 PO tid, increase as needed by 50 mg every four days, max 400 mg/day [50,100,150,300 mg].

-Bupropion (Wellbutrin) Initially: 100 mg PO bid, increase to 100 mg PO tid after 4 days prn; max 450 mg/day [75,100 mg].

-Fluoxetine (Prozac) 20 mg PO qd up to 80 mg day (divided doses) [20 mg].

-Doxepin (Sinequan) 75-150 mg PO qhs or 25-50 mg PO qd/tid, max 300 mg/day. [10,25,50,75,100,150 mg].**OR**

-Amitriptyline (Elavil, Endep) 25 mg PO tid **OR** 75 mg PO qhs, max 150 mg/day [10,25,50,85,100,150 mg].

-Protriptyline (Vivactil) 5-10 mg PO tid/qid, max 60 mg/day [5,10 mg].

MAO inhibitors

-Tranylcypromine (Parnate) 10 mg PO tid, max 60 mg/day [10 mg].

-Phenelzine (Nardil) Initially: 15 mg PO tid, increase rapidly (as tolerated to 60 mg daily) max 90 mg/day [15 mg]. Maintenance 15-30 mg daily.

BIPOLAR DISORDER

-Lithium 300 mg PO tid, adjust dose to blood level of 1.0 to 1.4 mg/L, before starting Lithium: CBC, thyroid function tests, blood urea nitrogen and serum creatine.

-Carbamazepine: Initially, 200 mg tid increase daily to 800-1200 mg/day; desired blood level of 8-12 mg/L.

ACUTE MANIC EPISODE

-Chlorpromazine (Thorazine) Initially: 25-50 mg PO tid or 25 mg IM every hour, may increase oral prn to 400 mg/day; IM up to 400 mg q4-6h until oral therapy is possible. [10,25,50,100,200 mg]

TREATMENT OF ANXIETY DISORDERS

GENERALIZED ANXIETY DISORDER

Benzodiazepines

-Alprazolam (Xanax) Initially: 0.25-0.5 mg PO tid, max 4 mg daily [0.25,0.5,1,2 mg].

-Diazepam (Valium) 2-10 mg PO tid/qid or for severe anxiety: 5-10 mg IM/IV q4h prn [2,5,10 mg].

-Lorazepam (Ativan) Initially: 1-3 mg PO q4-8h [0.5,1,2 mg].

Tricyclic Antidepressants

-Imipramine (Tofranil) 50-150 mg PO qhs, max 200 mg/day [10,25,50 mg].

-Doxepin (Sinequan) Initially: 25-50 mg PO qd, increase as needed to 75-150 mg qd or 25-50 mg PO bid/tid max 300 mg/day. [10,25,50,75,100,150 mg].

-Trazodone

PANIC DISORDER

Benzodiazepines

-Clonazepam (Klonopin) 0.5-2 mg PO qhs. [0.5,1,2 mg].

-Alprazolam (Xanax) Initially: 0.5 mg PO tid, increase prn by 0.5-1 mg/day doses up to 10 mg daily have been used [0.25,0.5,1,2 mg].

-Chlordiazepoxide (Librium) 5-25 mg PO tid/qid [5,10,25 mg].

-Diazepam (Valium) 2-10 mg PO tid/qid [2,5,10 mg].

Tricyclics

-Imipramine (Tofranil) 25-75 mg PO qhs or 25 mg PO qd/bid, max 200 mg/day [10,25,50 mg].

-Desipramine (Norpramin) 25-75 mg PO qhs, max 300 mg/day [10,25,50,75,100 mg].

-Nortriptyline (Pamelor) 25 mg PO qd/tid, max 150 mg/day [10,25,75 mg].

MAO Inhibitors

-Phenelzine (Nardil) 15 mg PO tid, max 90 mg/day [15 mg].

Other Agents

-Trazodone (Desyrel) 100 mg PO tid, max 450 mg/day [50,100,150,300 mg].

-Propranolol 10 mg PO qid increase daily to desired effect. Usual effective dose 40-160 mg/day. [10,20,40,60,80,90 mg].

POST TRAUMATIC STRESS DISORDER

Tricyclics

-Imipramine (Tofranil) 50-150 mg PO qhs, max 200 mg/day [10,25,50 mg].

Benzodiazepines

-Alprazolam (Xanax) Initially: 0.5 mg PO tid, may increase by 1 mg daily to 4 mg/day [0.25,0.5,1,2 mg].

-Oxazepam (Serax) 10-30 mg PO tid/qid. [10,15,30 mg].

-Lorazepam (Ativan) 1-3 mg PO q4-8h [0.5,1,2 mg].

Other Agents

-Buspirone (BuSpar) Initially: 5 mg PO tid, increase prn by 5 mg every 3 days to a max of 60 mg daily. [5,10 mg].

-Propranolol 20 mg PO tid increase to desired effect. Usual dosage 60-160 mg/day. [10,20,40,60,80,90 mg].

MAO Inhibitors

-Phenelzine (Nardil) 15 mg PO tid, max 90 mg/day [15 mg].

OBSESSIVE COMPULSIVE DISORDER

Cyclic Antidepressants:

-Clomipramine (Anafranil) Initially: 25 mg PO qd increase as tolerated to 100 mg/day (over 2 weeks), then increase over next two weeks to 250 mg daily [25,50,70].

-Fluoxetine (Prozac) 20 mg PO qd up to 80 mg day in divided doses [20 mg].

-Sertraline (Zoloft) 50-200 mg PO day (divided doses). [50,100 mg].

-Alprazolam (Xanax) 0.25-0.5 mg PO tid [0.25,0.5,1,2 mg].

-Tranylcypromine (Parnate) 10 mg PO bid, max 60 mg/day [10 mg]

AGORAPHOBIA

Tricyclics

-Amitriptyline (Elavil, Endep) 25 mg PO tid **or** 75 mg PO qhs, max 150 mg/day [10,25,50,85,100,150 mg].

-Doxepin (Sinequan) 25-75 mg PO qhs or 25 mg tid, max 300 mg/day [10,25,50,75,100,150 mg].

-Imipramine (Tofranil) 25-75 mg PO qhs, max 200 mg/day [10,25,50 mg].

-Trazodone 300 mg daily [50,100,150,300 mg].

-Sertraline (Zoloft) 50-200 mg daily [50,100 mg]

Benzodiazepines

-Alprazolam (Xanax) Initially: 0.5 mg PO tid, increase prn by 0.5-1 mg daily (doses up to 10 mg daily have been used) [0.25,0.5,1,2 mg].

-Chlordiazepoxide (Librium) 5-25 mg PO tid/qid [5,10,25 mg].

-Diazepam (Valium) 2-10 mg PO tid/qid [2,5,10 mg].

Other Agents

-Propranolol 20-40 mg before exposure to feared stimuli [10,20,40,60,80,90 mg].

SOCIAL PHOBIA

Beta Blockers

-Propranolol 20-40 mg before exposure to feared stimuli [10,20,40,60,80,90 mg].

MAO Inhibitors

-Phenelzine (Nardil) 15 mg PO tid, max 90 mg/day [15 mg].

-Tranylcypromine (Parnate) 10 mg PO bid, max 60 mg/day [10 mg].

Benzodiazepines

-Alprazolam (Xanax) 2-8 mg daily (divided doses). [0.25,0.5,1,2 mg].

TREATMENT OF PSYCHOTIC AND SUBSTANCE USE DISORDERS

SCHIZOPHRENIA

Antipsychotics

-Chlorpromazine (Thorazine) Initially: 10-25 mg PO qd/tid, increase prn up to 600 mg/day [10,25,50,100,200 mg].

-Trifluoperazine (Stelazine) 1-2 mg IM q4-6h or Initially: 2-5 mg PO bid, increase prn to 15-20 mg daily; max, 40 mg daily [1,2,5,10 mg].

-Thioridazine (Mellaril) Initially: 50-100 mg PO tid, increase prn to a max of 800 mg/day. [10,15,20,50,100,150,200 mg].

If Refractory:

-Clozapine (Clozaril) Initially 25 mg PO qd/tid, increase by 25 mg daily to 300-450 mg daily, if needed may be increase up to 900 mg daily. [25,100 mg]

SCHIZOPHRENIFORM DISORDER

Antipsychotics

-Chlorpromazine (Thorazine) Initially 10-25 mg PO qd/tid, increase prn up to 600 mg/day [10,25,50,100,200 mg].

-Trifluoperazine (Stelazine) Initially 1-2 mg IM q4-6h or 2-5 mg PO bid, increase prn up to 15-20 mg daily; max 40 mg daily [1,2,5,10 mg].

-Haloperidol (Haldol) 2-5 mg IM q4-8h prn (may be repeated as soon as 1 hr if needed) or 0.5-5 mg PO tid, up to 100 mg/day. [0.5,1,2,5,10,20 mg].

-Thiothixene (Navane) 4 mg IM q6-12h max 30 mg/day or 2-5 mg PO qid, max 60 mg/day [1,2,5,10,20 mg].

Benzodiazepines (anxiety or agitation):

-Clonazepam (Klonopin) 0.5-2 mg PO qhs [0.5,1,2 mg].

-Diazepam (Valium) 2-10 mg PO tid/qid. [2,5,10 mg].

-Lorazepam (Ativan) 1-3 mg PO q4-8h [0.5,1,2 mg].

Other Agents

-Lithium 300 mg PO tid, adjust dose to blood level of 1.0 to 1.4 mg/L.

SCHIZOAFFECTIVE DISORDER

Antipsychotics

-Trifluoperazine (Stelazine) 1-2 mg IM q4-6h or 2-5 mg PO bid, increase prn to 15-20 mg daily [1,2,5,10 mg].

-Thioridazine (Mellaril) 50-200 mg PO tid, max 800 mg/day [10,15,25,50,100,150,200 mg].

Antidepressants

-Fluoxetine (Prozac) 20 mg PO qd up to 80 mg day in divided doses [20 mg].

-Trazodone (Desyrel) Initially 50 mg PO tid, may be increase by 50 mg every 4 days to a max of 400 mg/day (outpatients) or 600 mg/day (outpatients). [50,100,150,300 mg].

-Bupropion (Wellbutrin) Initially 100 mg PO bid, increase to 100 mg PO tid after 4 days prn, max 450 mg/day, 150 mg (single dose) [75,100 mg].

Tricyclics

-Amitriptyline (Elavil, Endep) Initially: 25 mg PO tid **OR** 75 mg PO qhs, increase prn to a max of 150 mg/day (outpatients) or 300 mg/day (inpatients). [10,25,50,85,100,150 mg].

-Amoxapine (Asendin) Initially 50 mg PO bid/tid, increase to 100 mg PO bid/tid slowly over 1 week, once patient has adjusted, may be given as 300 mg PO qhs, max 400 mg/day, 300 mg/single dose [25,50,100,150 mg].

-Doxepin (Sinequan) Initially 25-50 mg PO tid or 75-150 mg PO qhs, increase prn to a max of 300 mg/day [10,25,50,75,100,150 mg].

Other Agents

-Lithium 300 mg PO tid, adjust dose to blood level of 1.0 to 1.4 mg/L.

-Carbamazepine: Initially, 200 mg tid increase daily to 800-1200 mg/day; desired blood level of 8-12 mg/L.

-Valproic acid may also be effective.

BRIEF REACTIVE PSYCHOSIS

Antipsychotics

-Chlorpromazine (Thorazine) Initially 10-25 mg PO bid/qid **OR** 25 mg slow IM every hour till patient is able to take oral form then 25-50 mg tid increase prn up to 600 mg/day. [10,25,50,100,200 mg].

-Trifluoperazine (Stelazine) 1-2 mg IM q4-6h or 2-5 mg PO bid, increase prn to 15-20 mg/day. [1,2,5,10 mg].

-Thioridazine (Mellaril) Initially: 50-100 mg PO tid, increase prn to a max of 800 mg/day [10,15,25,50,100,150,200 mg].

ORGANIC DELUSIONAL SYNDROME

Antipsychotics

-Treat underlying cause

-Chlorpromazine (Thorazine) Initially: 10-25 mg PO bid/tid or 25 mg slow IM q1-4h till oral therapy can be initiated, then 25 mg PO tid, increase prn up to 800 mg/day. [10,25,50,100,200 mg]

-Trifluoperazine (Stelazine) 1-2 mg IM q4-6h or 2-5 mg PO bid [1,2,5,10 mg].

-Thioridazine (Mellaril) Initially: 50-100 mg PO tid, increase prn to a max of 800 mg/day. [10,15,25,50,100,150,200 mg].

In Dementia Patients:

-Haloperidol (Haldol) 0.5-2 mg PO daily. [0.5,1,2,5,10,20 mg].

ALCOHOL WITHDRAWAL

Treatment:

-Chlordiazepoxide (Librium) 50-100 mg PO/IM/IV q2-6h (300 mg/d) [5,10,25 mg].**OR**

-Diazepam 10 mg PO tid/qid or 2-20 mg IM/IV q4-8h [2,5,10 mg].

-Clorazepate dipotassium 30 mg PO tid (1st day), 15 mg PO tid (2nd day), 5 mg PO qid (3rd day), 5 mg PO tid (4th day), then reduce prn till able to discontinue.

-Oxazepam (Serax) 15-30 mg PO tid, [10,15,30 mg]

-Carbamazepine (Tegretol) Initially, 100 mg PO bid, increase by 200 mg daily to 800 mg day.

-Mesoridazine (Serentil) Initially: 25 mg PO bid, increase prn to a max of 200 mg daily [10,25,50,100].

Delirium Tremens

-Chlordiazepoxide (Librium) 10 mg slow IV push or PO, repeat q4-6h prn agitation or tremor x 24h, max 500 mg/d. Then give 50-100 mg PO q6h prn agitation or tremor [5,10,25 mg].

-Diazepam (Valium) 2-20 mg IV/IM q3-4h. [2,5,10 mg].

Vitamins

-Magnesium sulfate 1 gm in 100 ml D5W over 2h qd.

-Multivitamin 1 amp IV then 1 tab PO qd.

-Thiamine 100 mg IM or IV qd x 3 days, then 100 mg PO qd

-Folate 1 mg IV, then 1 mg PO qd.

-Pyridoxine 100 mg IV/PO qd [10,25,50,100,250,500 mg].

INSOMNIA

Benzodiazepines

- Flurazepam (Dalmane)- 15-30 mg PO qhs [15,30 mg].
- Oxazepam (Serax) - 15-30 mg PO qhs [10,15,30 mg].
- Temazepam (Restoril)- 15-30 mg PO qhs [15,30 mg].
- Triazolam (Halcion) - 0.125-0.25 mg PO qhs [0.125,0.25 mg].

Non-benzodiazepines

- Zolpidem (Ambien) - 10 mg PO qhs [10 mg].

INDEX

REGISTRATION CARD AND ORDER FORM

Submission of this form (with or without ordering) entitles you to receive FREE drug updates, revision announcements, catalogs and discounts on our publications.

Current Clinical Strategies, Prescription Writer Computer Program
Prescription Writing System & Record Manager. Produces legible prescriptions in seconds, and keeps an updated list of each patient's medications. Includes a database of over 1500 dosages. Installs on any IBM computer; dot matrix or laser printer. No special paper required, Rx paper included. Windows required. Available 11/30/94.
Please circle one: 5¼ 3½ inch diskettes #___x $55.00

Current Clinical Strategies, Physician's Drug Resource (available 8/15/94) #___x $8.75

Current Clinical Strategies, Practice Parameters in Primary Care Medicine (8/3094) #___x $12.75

Handbook of Anesthesia
Mark Ezekiel, MD #___x $8.75

Manual of HIV/AIDS Therapy
Laurence Peiperl, MD #___x $8.75

Current Clinical Strategies, MEDICINE, Paul D. Chan, MD NEW 1994 edition #___x $8.75

Current Clinical Strategies, GYNECOLOGY & OBSTETRICS, NEW 1994 edition #___x $10.75

Current Clinical Strategies, PEDIATRICS, NEW 1994 edition #___x $8.75

FAMILY MEDICINE, NEW 1995 edition
Pediatrics, Medicine, Gynecology, Obstetrics #___x $26.25

DIAGNOSTIC HISTORY & PHYSICAL EXAMINATION in MEDICINE #___x $8.75

OUTPATIENT MEDICINE #___x $8.75

CRITICAL CARE MEDICINE #___x $8.75

PSYCHIATRY #___x $8.75

HANDBOOK OF PSYCHIATRIC DRUG THERAPY #___x $8.75

Current Clinical Strategies, SURGERY #___x$8.75

Shipping and Handling, add $2.00 per book $ _______

Total _____

Please complete reverse side.

Prices are in US dollars. Other countries, send equivalent amount in foreign check. Prices and availability subject to change without notice.

Order by Phone: 1-714-965-9400 (add $1.50 COD charge per order; a bill will be sent with order)

Order by Mail. Send order & check payable to:

Current Clinical Strategies Publishing
9550 Warner Ave, Suite 213
Fountain Valley, Ca USA 92708-2822

Return Address: ______________________________

____

____

Phone Number: (_______)______________________________

Is this book sold at your local medical book store? ___ yes ___ no
Name, address and phone number of bookstore that does not carry our books:

____

____

____

Receive $8.75 off your order if this book is not available in your local bookstore. Receive discount by enclosing a bookstore business card signed by the bookstore manager stating that they are out of stock. Take $8.75 off total.
Enclose the cover of your old edition and receive $2.00 off your order when you purchase the new edition.

Comments:
We appreciate your comments -- good and bad -- about our books and software.

Suggested additions, problems or criticisms:

____

____

____

____

REGISTRATION CARD AND ORDER FORM

Submission of this form (with or without ordering) entitles you to receive FREE drug updates, revision announcements, catalogs and discounts on our publications.

Current Clinical Strategies, Prescription Writer Computer Program
Prescription Writing System & Record Manager. Produces legible prescriptions in seconds, and keeps an updated list of each patient's medications. Includes a database of over 1500 dosages. Installs on any IBM computer; dot matrix or laser printer. No special paper required, Rx paper included. Windows required. Available 11/30/94.
Please circle one: 5¼ 3½ inch diskettes #___x $55.00

Current Clinical Strategies, #___x $8.75
Physician's Drug Resource (available 8/15/94)

Current Clinical Strategies, Practice Parameters #___x $12.75
in Primary Care Medicine (8/3094)

Handbook of Anesthesia #___x $8.75
Mark Ezekiel, MD

Manual of HIV/AIDS Therapy #___x $8.75
Laurence Peiperl, MD

Current Clinical Strategies, #___x $8.75
MEDICINE, Paul D. Chan, MD NEW 1994 edition

Current Clinical Strategies, #___x $10.75
GYNECOLOGY & OBSTETRICS, NEW 1994 edition

Current Clinical Strategies, #___x $8.75
PEDIATRICS, NEW 1994 edition

FAMILY MEDICINE, NEW 1995 edition #___x $26.25
Pediatrics, Medicine, Gynecology, Obstetrics

DIAGNOSTIC HISTORY & PHYSICAL #___x $8.75
EXAMINATION in MEDICINE

OUTPATIENT MEDICINE #___x $8.75

CRITICAL CARE MEDICINE #___x $8.75

PSYCHIATRY #___x $8.75

HANDBOOK OF PSYCHIATRIC DRUG THERAPY #___x $8.75

Current Clinical Strategies, #___x$8.75
SURGERY

Shipping and Handling, add $2.00 per book $ _______

Total _____

Please complete reverse side.

Prices are in US dollars. Other countries, send equivalent amount in foreign check. Prices and availability subject to change without notice.

Order by Phone: 1-714-965-9400 (add $1.50 COD charge per order; a bill will be sent with order)

Order by Mail. Send order & check payable to:

Current Clinical Strategies Publishing
9550 Warner Ave, Suite 213
Fountain Valley, Ca USA 92708-2822

Return Address: ______________________________

____

____

Phone Number: (_______)______________________________

Is this book sold at your local medical book store? ___ yes ___ no
Name, address and phone number of bookstore that does not carry our books:

____

____

____

Receive $8.75 off your order if this book is not available in your local bookstore. Receive discount by enclosing a bookstore business card signed by the bookstore manager stating that they are out of stock. Take $8.75 off total.
Enclose the cover of your old edition and receive $2.00 off your order when you purchase the new edition.

Comments:
We appreciate your comments -- good and bad -- about our books and software.

Suggested additions, problems or criticisms:

____

____

____

____

REGISTRATION CARD AND ORDER FORM

Submission of this form (with or without ordering) entitles you to receive FREE drug updates, revision announcements, catalogs and discounts on our publications.

Current Clinical Strategies, Prescription Writer Computer Program Prescription Writing System & Record Manager. Produces legible prescriptions in seconds, and keeps an updated list of each patient's medications. Includes a database of over 1500 dosages. Installs on any IBM computer; dot matrix or laser printer. No special paper required, Rx paper included. Windows required. Available 11/30/94. Please circle one: 5¼ 3½ inch diskettes	#___x $55.00
Current Clinical Strategies, Physician's Drug Resource (available 8/15/94)	#___x $8.75
Current Clinical Strategies, Practice Parameters in Primary Care Medicine (8/3094)	#___x $12.75
Handbook of Anesthesia Mark Ezekiel, MD	#___x $8.75
Manual of HIV/AIDS Therapy Laurence Peiperl, MD	#___x $8.75
Current Clinical Strategies, MEDICINE, Paul D. Chan, MD NEW 1994 edition	#___x $8.75
Current Clinical Strategies, GYNECOLOGY & OBSTETRICS, NEW 1994 edition	#___x $10.75
Current Clinical Strategies, PEDIATRICS, NEW 1994 edition	#___x $8.75
FAMILY MEDICINE, NEW 1995 edition Pediatrics, Medicine, Gynecology, Obstetrics	#___x $26.25
DIAGNOSTIC HISTORY & PHYSICAL EXAMINATION in MEDICINE	#___x $8.75
OUTPATIENT MEDICINE	#___x $8.75
CRITICAL CARE MEDICINE	#___x $8.75
PSYCHIATRY	#___x $8.75
HANDBOOK OF PSYCHIATRIC DRUG THERAPY	#___x $8.75
Current Clinical Strategies, SURGERY	#___x$8.75
Shipping and Handling, add $2.00 per book	$ _______
	Total _____

Please complete reverse side.

Prices are in US dollars. Other countries, send equivalent amount in foreign check. Prices and availability subject to change without notice.

Order by Phone: 1-714-965-9400 (add $1.50 COD charge per order; a bill will be sent with order)

Order by Mail. Send order & check payable to:

Current Clinical Strategies Publishing
9550 Warner Ave, Suite 213
Fountain Valley, Ca USA 92708-2822

Return Address: ______________________________

____

____

Phone Number: (_______)______________________

Is this book sold at your local medical book store? ___ yes ___ no
Name, address and phone number of bookstore that does not carry our books:

____

____

____

Receive $8.75 off your order if this book is not available in your local bookstore. Receive discount by enclosing a bookstore business card signed by the bookstore manager stating that they are out of stock. Take $8.75 off total.

Enclose the cover of your old edition and receive $2.00 off your order when you purchase the new edition.

Comments:

We appreciate your comments -- good and bad -- about our books and software.

Suggested additions, problems or criticisms:

____

____

____

____